My Breast Cancer Journey:

12 Life Lessons it Taught Me

From Triple Negative to Very Positive

Grace Nolan

Table of Contents

The 12 Life Lessons

These are boxed within the text and are reflections and realisations that stood out for me during a really hard time and helped me get through. They are things I already knew but I had to be reminded that it's not enough to be aware of them, I needed to put them into practise and actually live them.

Dedication

To my husband John with love –
I couldn't have made it through without you.

Foreword

To anyone who has had a diagnosis of breast cancer, I can only tell you what I'm going through. I hope it helps you and that it gives you a bit more strength on your own journey or even one tip to alleviate some of your discomfort and fear. Keep in mind though that most of the time, if not all of it, my head is fuzzy and foggy and I can't think straight – apparently, it's called "Chemo Brain" – it's real, I can vouch for that because I've always loved having a clear mind – looks like I finally have to experience what it's like not to have one and to have to see my way through a very cloudy patch and hope it's just temporary. "Temporary" – it's the only thing that pushes me on – that this will be over and that I'm still standing at the end of it.

It's hard for me to believe that if it hadn't been for the decision to try acupuncture for the first time in my life, I most likely would not be here today telling this story. I'm going to be very honest about it all. It's the story of a very ordinary, healthy person who, out of nowhere and without any real family history – apart from one aunt who is still living in her nineties, is suddenly faced with a diagnosis of the worst type of breast cancer. Luckily, because of those acupuncture sessions which I was having to help with arthritis, the cancer was discovered early.

Everyone's experience is unique and it's important to remember that there are many different chemo treatments with a wide variety of medications used and that each treatment is tailored to the individual. Most people don't have allergic reactions to the combination of drugs as I did: I had an aversion to food and drink especially in the first weeks of each treatment, whereas some patients were eating and drinking during their actual hospital sessions without any adverse effects at all. I have always been extremely sensitive to chemicals and have avoided taking any medicines because of the side effects they have on me.

Despite all this, I hope my experience helps you even in a small way to deal with what you are going through or helps you to understand what someone else is going through. So, I will call you my friend or perhaps even my sister (or brother) and I'll lead the way forward to make the path a little easier for you. Everyone has their own story to tell with their own hopes and dreams. This is mine and I welcome you as you walk with me.

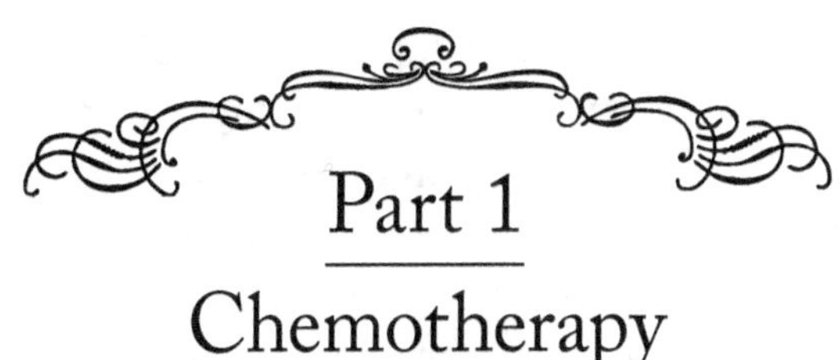

Part 1

Chemotherapy

17 / 12 / 2018 Monday 8.15 am

My first Chemo session. I'm scared. I don't want to feel scared but I am. Hospital has never been for me; it's always been for someone else – Mum, Dad, my husband, John, and I've been the physically strong and healthy one by their side, worrying about them. I've never been the sick one for anything serious and I'm not the sick one now. Except for the tenderness in the right breast which had surgery on it two weeks ago I feel perfectly fine. The three incisions have been healing really well.

This is a completely different experience for me. Looking quickly around the oncology ward I'm surprised to see how busy it is – one huge room full of big chairs with men and women sitting in them with drips in their arms and nurses administering medications and taking down notes and results. I'm in a smaller narrow room off the bigger one with only four chairs in it and a kitchenette right in front. Everything is designed to make things softer, more comfortable, and not as terrifying as it really is but the truth is that all of it is horrendous. I don't dwell on any of it and I try not to notice anything much because I know that's the best way for me in this circumstance. I feel dazed and out of it and that helps me to cope, so I don't force myself to shake out of it, I give into it instead. I try to catch the eye of the two people either side of me – one woman a few years older than me and a woman much younger than me. The older woman turns towards the wall and doesn't want to be greeted and the younger one appears to be asleep. I just want to smile at them and give them some encouragement and maybe receive some too but none of that is forthcoming though it would be really great. The nurses on the other hand are beautiful, smiling and friendly so it takes a bit of the edge off my nervousness. Erin, one of the nurses, asks me many questions and notes down many things and I ask her when my last session will be, "That way I can work towards a goal," I say to her. "When I know what the end date is, I can cross off days on the calendar and feel better knowing the final day is closer and closer." She tells me that's a great idea and is very happy that I'm approaching the Chemo in a positive way and hurries off to find out the exact date of my final treatment.

Two nurses work together to get things ready for me – a couple of tiny vials with liquid in them, a tablet I have to take under the tongue, the intravenous needle into the back of my hand ready for the Chemotherapy.

I've opted to try the head freezing cap which means hopefully I won't lose all my hair, but it's hard to find the right fit. There's lots of pulling and tugging and starting again by the two nurses but they're finally satisfied that they've got it right. It's uncomfortable but I can manage it. I'm sitting on a big padded armchair that can extend into a type of bed if I need to lie back, and even though it's Summertime and very hot outside I'm wearing fleecy winter clothes and Erin, the nurse who is to look after me has covered me in a thick blanket. This is because the freezing cap is going to make me feel extremely cold. I've been told I may not be able to endure it and I can ask for it to be stopped at any time. I want to give it a go as I'd rather not be completely bald but this is a relatively new technique and by the sounds of it, a bit hit and miss. My head starts to feel horribly cold but my husband, John is holding my hand and asking if I'm all right and that makes me be all right. The clock is facing me high up on the wall and finally fifteen minutes are up and I've done what I've been told is the worst part.

Now they start the drugs – I didn't know that hadn't started. After a few minutes or less than that, I suddenly start to feel terrible in the stomach – the belly region – really terrible. I tap the nurse on the back – she is seeing to the patient next to me. I can hardly reach her, then suddenly I have a shocking pain in my lower back so bad I can hardly breathe. "What level of pain are you feeling from one to ten?" asks Erin. "Nine," I groan, and unbelievably I *am* groaning - involuntarily. Within seconds a heat pack is administered and I think it's that which has given me relief. (I don't know till weeks later that a sedative was administered – pumped into the drip.) It was terrible but quick and the pain is gone and now I'm feeling very drowsy and I zonk out for most of the day and night – which I very much prefer and feel grateful for. We're still at the hospital - I remember John feeding me red jelly and I can hardly open my mouth but I like the taste of it so I try to suck it in. Then I have a few bites of the little sandwiches and I can feed myself the tiny tub of ice-cream with the little wooden paddle – what a luxury! I remember my oncology specialist talking to me but not what she said.

I remember being glad it was over, the cap lifted off my head, me a bit unsteady on my feet and holding onto John's arm. And we're in the car and heading home!

The five hours of treatment have finally finished as well as the extra hour and a half of waiting in the middle of the dose, after my bad reaction to the drugs. When I ring my sister, Maria, and my brother Vincent, I feel like I've achieved something: "I'm okay – just feeling dazed but I'm all right. I can't remember anything at the moment – did I already say that?" I've had my first Chemo treatment so I can start marking the days off the calendar. This is the beginning of the end of the treatment but nothing is making much sense to me. "I feel stupid that I can't remember the right words – they do say it's called 'chemo brain'. It's horrible! I feel fuzzy in the head," I say to Maria.

My sister sounds relieved that the first session is over. She's been anxiously waiting to hear from me. "Sis, are you kidding!" Maria says fervently, "You're fighting the biggest enemy known to man – that's killing off millions of people! It's enough for you just to survive it. Look after yourself and don't worry about anything else." I'm lucky to have such a great sister. My brother and sister-in-law, Lorrie, are equally encouraging, attentive and caring after my quick call to them. "Just get better Sis," says Vincent, "I've had the candle going for you," and I know he's been praying for me and been really worried about me. But I can't help feeling foolish as I'm not able to articulate a clear sentence and some of my words are coming out distorted. It's all a bit frightening. I won't let it overpower me, though. I am quite determined about that!

LIFE LESSON:
ALLOW YOURSELF TO FEEL SCARED

So often we feel, or are made to feel foolish or cowardly for being frightened but usually there's very good reason for it. I've learnt that it's okay to feel scared – terrified even – how can you not feel scared in the face of this? You have to give yourself permission to experience the fear; feel it and acknowledge it. The key is not to let it take over.

6.00pm

I'm still stunned when I think about it: me having cancer! It doesn't seem to go together at all. It's a word I've always chosen not to say – something I don't think about – banish from my thoughts. But it has sneaked in unseen, unnoticed, like a thief in the night stealing away my good health and my peace of mind. Maybe I've been too complacent. It's shaken up my whole world and I don't want it to. I refuse to give it importance for to do that would give it power over me. I don't want to fight it for to fight it means I am setting myself up for the possibility of losing and I have no intention of losing. I think maybe the thing to do is to release it. I'm trying to find the message in it, if there is one – take the message, accept the lesson and let the rest go. I release it now out of my body, and out of my life forever and I'll try not to fall into the same patterns of thinking and ways of living because they are what brought me here and obviously something about that didn't work. I feel this instinctively.

Changes need to happen if I am to be well – changes in thinking and behaviour. Loving myself more, not putting myself and my feelings last as I've always done, paying attention to my feelings, not allowing myself to feel pressured or stressed into doing things I don't want to do. Overworking, over caring, overdoing – this is the pattern of my life and it needs to change. I want to remain caring and loving because that's the most important part of me, but not overdoing it at my expense every time. Doing everything in a loving way is vital, even when drawing away from a friendship or relationship, but not allowing others to dictate and manipulate and bully.

This high thinking is well and good but the truth is: I'm puzzled and confused and a bit dazed. What will this mean for me and my husband and for my family? I don't know what any of it means. What a strange thing to happen! Yet I know thousands of people battle with cancer every day. I don't like it; I don't want it. How did this happen? Did I let this happen? I don't want to be afraid. I refuse to be afraid. While I'm making this stand, I'm quivering inside - but just enough to make firm my resolve.

I've just decided I will not treat this as I was treating it before - as an unseen enemy that has crept in, and stealthily and slyly taken up abode unbeknown to me. I will see this as an awakening that brings me closer to a fuller understanding of myself. I will find the blessing in it for there must be one – all my long, life experience has taught me this about everything – even the worst of circumstances. For once I won't let fear rule. I will stand firm. I will be brave. I will call on every ounce of courage within me.

Some people might feel crushed, shocked, sorrowful, weary, overwhelmed, defeated and I feel all those things but most of all, and stronger than everything else – I feel determined – completely determined to get through.

LIFE LESSON:
DECIDE TO BE BRAVE

You will be amazed at how much inner strength you have, both mental and emotional. Call on all your reserves of resilience and determination. Make a conscious decision that no matter how scared you are, you will face whatever is necessary with courage. Be brave for yourself and for those who love you.

18/12/2018 Tuesday

My first day after Chemo! I slept only three hours last night but felt restful anyway. I felt wide awake at 1.30am and I couldn't sleep after that. I may have dozed a bit. Considering everything, I've had a pretty good day. I feel all right and have done many things: I've written out Christmas cards, sent texts, sent emails, read a little, made porridge, fried up the left over pasta for lunch, heated up the soup for tea – all delicious food Maria made for us. I've taken all my tablets this morning and been to the local doctor's clinic to have my platelets injection – a one-and-a-half hour wait after a mix-up – of course! But I feel okay. John and I just went for a walk – slowly, but all fine. I put my hands in my pockets to hide my black-painted nails when we pass others along the way. The black nail polish apparently helps prevent the nails from dropping off because of the Chemo so I've put it on my fingernails and toenails with quite a lot of difficulty as I've never had much practise with nail polish before now.

I spoke to Kelly on the phone, a hospital receptionist confirming an appointment. I've spoken to Maria and Vincent and Lorrie, on the phone too so I feel happy, and satisfied that I've done quite a bit. I'm pleased that I've still got all my hair. I've had a few symptoms: dry mouth, hot soles of the feet and palms of the hands, beginning of ulcers in my mouth, sore gums when I bit on a piece of pane di casa bread, breathlessness and a very small voice but it's all okay.

I've also received cards, texts and emails today from my friends, all full of love and support. Overall, I feel okay – relieved but still a bit nervous – not knowing what the day will bring. My heart has been beating faster than usual. We had morning tea with Maria – she made cupcakes for me to celebrate getting over my first major hurdle.

I still have a racing heart. It's hard to relax. I feel a bit tense, as though everything could easily spiral out of control such as pain, vomiting etc. but I need to get off that track. I'm lucky, very lucky to have John and people around me who love me.

19/12/2018 Wednesday

This morning not so good.

Felt nauseous after breakfast – had a tablet to combat it. Felt teary and cried. I hate this feeling. John sat next to me and we both cried a bit. I feel low in energy today.

Ulcers in my mouth feel like they want to break out. There is a horrible chemical taste in my mouth too. I have been doing my mouthwashes as instructed by the nurses and the manual I've been given.

My sister has discovered that she needs to have a gastroscopy. John has taken her so I'll be alone for a few hours – a little bit scary but not too bad. I'm trying to sweep the floor and tidy up a bit. I have spoken to Vincent and Lorrie on the phone. Today I've also spoken to some other very dear long-time friends, Rozanne and Janine as well as Dzintra and Francis who are like family – all brief calls but it's been a big phone call day. I've had messages from my niece, Grace, and my nephews, Sandy and Paul and I can feel the love and support so strongly from all of them, especially by the fact that most of them get all the updates from my sister and she relays their messages so it takes all the pressure off me. I love all my family, more than I can say – and this includes friends. And while I'm reflecting on this, I'm thinking seriously that I might have overdone it a bit as I'm feeling quite weary and worn out. But they're good thoughts and feelings of being looked after and cared about which I know is a huge blessing in my life.

I felt headachy this morning and was flushed in the cheeks – I had no temperature though. I was thinking that I would like to wash my hair but knew it was better to wait a week as I've been told to do if I want some to stay on after all that cold cap hassle which lengthens the Chemo procedure by a couple of hours. I only slept three hours during the night at first. Slept again a bit after a break in the middle. I have been trying to stay positive although my feet feel very hot.

20/12/2018 Thursday

Aching limbs! So sore I can hardly walk. Everything hurts. This is horrible! I've put the washing on though. I've done three days of Chemo already – three days closer to the end of the treatment. I'm crossing the days off the calendar. I've decided I'll only cross the day off after it's absolutely finished, that is, the next day. I don't want to count my chickens – I've already had a taste of how quickly things can change before the day is finished. My Temperature: 37.98

21/12/2018 Friday

Nearly ended up in hospital today. Feeling ghastly. Everything hurts. Don't like food or drink but trying hard to keep it up – or should I say down. Luckily Kristen, the day oncology nurse phoned to check on how I was going. She told me to phone my specialist, Professor Emma Rosewall. She also told me I needed to take more tablets: pain killers, anti-inflammatory, and more anti-nausea pills. She says things should get better. I truly hope so.

22/12/2018 Saturday

My Temperature: 36.4 this morning. Got two to three good hours of sleep. Awake after that – dozing occasionally. Burning genitals back and front. Had to get up at 4.50am – kidneys so painful throughout the night but now impossible to put up with. Two anti-inflammatory tablets immediately – pain settling down after a few minutes but the itching is demonic. John has gone to the supermarket for cranberry juice at 7.10am. He is worried and doesn't know what to do. I feel a bit better but he says I look much paler than other days. I've decided to tick off days on the calendar instead of crossing them off so it's more positive – have ticked off five days. My dear brother Vincent, who lives in Queensland has told me he will phone me every day while I'm having the cancer treatments and I've decided to tick off each day after I've spoken to him – that way I can look forward to two things, the phone call and the tick on the calendar.

The worst day of all so far. A swelling on the right side of my throat. A swelling on the left side is the worst. Pain galore in joints and legs. Tired, headachy, dazed; reading vision not good; mouth tastes like I've drunk a bottle of poison. I feel that I can't make it through no matter how strong I'm trying to be. There is nothing - no words at all to describe this state my body is in and how dreadfully sick I feel. I don't want to be weak and silly but even with all my determination to remain positive I'm crumbling mentally under the huge pressure of being so sick and helpless. I physically can't withstand it and I strongly feel that if I'm going to die, I want to die at home. My body is shouting: "Don't ever dare do this again!"

If I survive this, I can't put my body through another round of Chemo because of the severe treatment-related symptoms I've been experiencing. I'm considering pulling out of it. One moment I think it's the right thing to do and the next moment I'm unsure.

Just as I'm thinking I won't have another treatment, Rozanne, a long-time friend says to me, "Grace, you've got to do this!" She says it quietly, firmly and definitely and I trust this because she is very in tune with things and she is not a person who ever forces her opinion or gives advice unless asked. She has just phoned and I've briefly stated in a tiny, teary voice that doesn't sound like me at all that I can't go on – that the Chemo is literally killing me. Later she doesn't remember saying this to me – I think it was divine intervention when I was at a crossroads. My closest family and friends all agree that I probably need to go on with the treatments no matter how bad they are because of the type of cancer I was diagnosed with – triple negative – one of the most aggressive types of breast cancer which spreads rapidly and doesn't respond to anything other than the most aggressive forms of treatment. At this stage it hasn't fully sunk in for me – it all feels very strange and unreal - as unreal as when I first received the diagnosis from my doctor.

Seven weeks earlier

1/11/2018 Thursday 2.10pm

Doctor Mark Frankel looks at the report on his computer. He cringes visibly and inadvertently puts both arms across his stomach as though it is causing him discomfort. He wasn't expecting this. I can see it's painful for him to read it. I wait a little while. "It's not good news, is it?" I say to spare him a bit. "The tests have shown there is a lump and it's cancer." It doesn't seem real to me at all and I don't even look at John, sitting beside me. "Is it serious?" I ask. (Looking back, I can see how this must have seemed a very stupid question) He looks at me with a pained look on his face. "It's breast cancer," he says. I still can't completely take it in and maybe it's better that way to let it wash off me. It doesn't seem real and I don't want it to be real. I don't know what all this means. Doctor Frankel is a very knowledgeable man who genuinely cares about his patients which sets him apart as an excellent G.P. – after all he is the one who has seen John through all his heart issues since 1990. He feels sorry for me. "You're going to have to endure surgery, Chemotherapy and Radiation Treatment," he says gently. Still not real. I don't know fully what it means, but at the back of my mind there are images of people who look like death, hooked up to machines, vomiting violently, and almost bald, with wisps of hair and sunken eyes. Oh God! I push these images away. I've never wanted to dwell on illness – don't make it real – just deal with it a step at a time until all is healed and throw everything you've got at it – use everything at your disposal – use every means of healing you have access to. "So, what's the next step?" I ask. "You'll have to undergo surgery to remove the lump and the other two small growths in the right breast," Doctor Frankel replies. "Put me onto the best person you know," I say in a very determined voice. Doctor Frankel gets straight onto the phone and calls someone at Cabrini Hospital. The appointment is set up. I am so impressed by this marvellous doctor of ours. He is a truly kind, intelligent and competent man. I feel I can trust his guidance and decisions.

John and I leave his office feeling grateful for his quick help. I still feel puzzled and unsure – and disbelieving: maybe there's been a mistake. Are the results correct?

28/11/2018 Wednesday morning

The morning of my afternoon breast surgery to remove the two cancerous lumps and the two benign growths is the most painful of all the experiences. I have to have two Hook Wires inserted into my right breast which are as excruciating as they sound and take a long time *to secure in the correct places. The ultrasound the nurses have just done shows that I need two as another growth has appeared since last time the ultrasound was done so they have to be sure to get everything. The arm I have to hold above my head is numb and aching to a terrible extent. After that I have to have another mammogram with the Hook Wires in and my legs buckle and I nearly faint from the pain. The nurse has to reposition things — she hadn't realised how painful it would be.*

The injection I have before all this, directly into the aureole of the breast is quick but extremely painful for a moment — so much so that I let out an involuntary scream. It surprises me and I apologise to the doctor. He says not to feel bad at all about a little scream because by this stage some women have slapped his face and uttered a few choice words and it is unusual I haven't done the same. I chuckle at this and appreciate the doctor's kindness and humour as he tries his best to help me relax while I lie on the narrow hospital table under the lights with a nurse beside me and another one near a big scanning machine I've just been under. The number of scans and tests before the operation is phenomenal — I'm being so well looked after but I'm not completely taking it in. I feel as though I'm in a disconcerting, bad dream.

The surgery goes really well and I'm told I am a good healer as the three incisions heal quickly and beautifully. I can't take full credit for that - I know a lot of it has to do with the great skill of Miss Julia Kirk, my wonderful surgeon.

23/12/2018 Sunday

I've had to phone my oncologist, Emma, again. She has told me to take the steroid tablet each day and wants to see me tomorrow. The tablet helps to calm down the allergies. Felt very sick for about three hours after tea. Ate a bit too much and a bit too hot and too cold. I've discovered it's this steroid tablet that makes me feel teary and nervous – they are its side effects for me but I need the tablets to control the side effects of the Chemo drugs which are worse.

24/12/2018 Monday

We're going to Cabrini Hospital to see Emma. She examines under my arms – there is still a slight rash visible – the other itchiness has subsided - thank God! I have two pages of notes to try to tell her how bad it has all been and I start to read them out.

Emma understands and fairly expects me to pull out of the program – there can be no doubt that the side-effects I've been experiencing are alarming. She is sympathetic and concerned and says I've had a severe allergic reaction to one of the Chemo drugs, Docetaxel. I suddenly realise that the extreme sickness I have been experiencing has not just been caused by the Chemo but has been compounded by the allergic reaction. Emma says she can't guarantee it won't happen again even with a different drug which she is going to replace it with called Epirubicin – the Cyclophosphamide will remain the same. It's frightening. All the drugs associated with Chemo sound like weed killers to me, but then cancer is like a noxious weed that, allowed to take root and grow unchecked, eventually strangles the life out of you. So, I suppose it's fitting that the medicines used to eradicate it should be called by those frightening names. I know that sometimes the so-called cure can kill the patient – it nearly killed Vincent three years ago: the dye that was injected into him before the heart stents could be put in gave him anaphylactic shock; it killed him twice and he had to be revived and ended up being written about in a medical journal. He actually went over to the other side for a while! I've asked him about it many times and each time he tells me about it he's very casual and never makes a big deal of it, while I'm left stunned and wanting to hear every detail. Some things were for him personally so he keeps those to himself but he does say, "It confirms that there's more – that without a shadow of a doubt there's more and it's better. It confirms that there's another life beyond this."

Emma leaves the decision entirely up to me, and John agrees with me that I can't go through another week like the last one.

I say to Emma, "If it was your mother sitting here in my place what would you advise her to do?" "I think I might say to her to give it one more try and you can stop at any moment," she says, with her head on one side and real empathy and feeling in her voice. But I know once the drug is in, they can't get it out and it starts wreaking havoc and then there is only pain management while the side-effects keep raging and my body which doesn't even feel like it's my own is desperately trying to hold on. I don't want to read the patient handouts I've been given. They're too clinical: they outline risks and side effects and all sorts of horrors that it's best not to know too much about or you begin wondering why you are agreeing to put yourself through this.

25/12/2018 Tuesday 5.48am Christmas morning.

This morning I have felt my most normal so far since the treatment. Throughout the night, though, I woke up in a sweat with the neck and arms of my night dress wet. It kept happening - I had to change four nighties but I feel okay.

John and I are spending Christmas day on our own. Firstly, I don't have the energy to be around lots of people and engage in conversation or even listen to it no matter how much I love them all. Secondly, I am wary of picking up any germs from anyone who might have a cold or sniffles which is hard to avoid when there are about twenty people including children at the family gathering.

12.15pm

My sister is sending over a Christmas lunch and it is dropped off at the door by my niece and nephew who are always kind and giving. It's so good to see their beautiful, smiling faces and experience their real concern for me. They have brought a basketful of goodies and gifts. I don't feel like eating anything but I can see the food looks delicious and has been made and delivered with so much love and thoughtfulness and I will certainly make an effort to taste what I can. Apart from that, John needs to eat and will enjoy the feast.

I'm going to tick off another day!

27/12/2018 Thursday

Finding it hard to sleep – have had two hours. Up and reading now at 1.30am – *The Narnia Chronicles* – lovely.

Have had a deep insight into one of the causes of this cancer problem when, Aslan, the magnificent lion and Divine figure in *Prince Caspian* says to Susan who is one of the children called to the land of Narnia:

> *"You have listened to fears, child, … Come, let me breathe on you. Forget them. Are you brave again?" "A little, Aslan," said Susan.*

I can say this to myself: "You have listened to fears, my girl. You have let them eat away at you, to diminish and deplete you. You have allowed despair to creep in. It's deadly for you. Let me breathe on you, my child. Are you brave again?"

"Be kinder to yourself - you know, the way you're kind to other people? Be kind like that to you."

"I don't know if I can do that."

"Well, you're going to have to try because if you keep on neglecting yourself and ignoring what you want, you'll end up in the same place – don't you see that otherwise you'll be repeating the same pattern? and when you do that, you'll get the same result."

28/12/2018 Friday

Had a heart scan today at Cabrini Hospital called a Gater Blood Pool Scan because of the necessary change in medication for Chemo. This replacement drug I'm now on, also one of those dubbed "red devil" because of its red colour and its horrendous, potential side effects, has more risk of damaging the heart. It's more reason for me to try and stay strong. The test didn't hurt – just imaging after blood was taken out and put back into my arm by Connor, a 6 foot 5 inch gentle giant who has squirted some radiation molecules into it. He made me feel at ease with his sense of humour underneath all that orange-red hair and beard. "Could you give me some warning before you take the blood," I ask, "I need to close my eyes so I don't see the needle, if that's all right." "That's fine!" he replies, "So do I! but I'll keep my eyes open this time." "I suppose as long as one of us can see what's going on, it'll be okay," I add with a chuckle. After that I'm sent to the waiting room to allow time for the molecules to travel before the scan is taken.

Met Jenny, a 75-year-old lady in the waiting room while the procedure was taking effect. "You Greek?" she asked, coming over tentatively and sitting next to me. "Italian," I answer. In this moment it makes no difference that I was born in Australia and have lived my whole life here except for one year when I was a child. "Ah, Italian!" she says and there is instant understanding between us – we are both from European backgrounds. She tells me she has a problem with her heart and her son is picking her up.

"What you have?" she asks. "Cancer," I say, "Breast cancer." "Oh!" up till now she has been quite animated but her face falls and she forgets about her own aches. I'm surprised. She feels incredibly sad for me. "My friend had the same," she says, "had Chemo – everything, then it came back after seven years. She died three years ago." "Oh dear!" I think to myself, "Another one of those horrible stories." Jenny continues unaware that this sort of information is not helpful to me. "We not take care of ourselves," she says, shaking her head in disapproval.

"We always have worry about family – this one, that one, the other one." "We need to look after ourselves," I say and she agrees. "Now we know but it too late!" she exclaims. "No, it's not too late," I say, looking directly at her. "It's never too late. We still have some good years – both of us." "You right! It never too late," she says in a slightly resigned voice.

We both have finally got it – it has taken us this long, I'm sixty and she's seventy-five and we both wish we had understood this properly long, long ago, instead of expending useless worry on countless unnecessary things. "Work! Pressure!" says Jenny, pushing her hands down to emphasise the extent of it. "Worry! Stress!" I add, "These four things are killers and lead to illness. We need to relax more," I say. We both agree. We have both independently come to the same realisation and now we both voice our thoughts. We are friends – we speak the same language.

I'm fast coming to the conclusion that like the Seven Deadly Sins in Religious belief: Pride, Gluttony, Covetousness, Envy, Lust, Sloth and Anger, there are seven deadly sins of cancer: worry, stress, pressure, overwork, grief, regret, remorse – and actually I think there's one more: guilt – negative, deadly things that eat away at us and take away our peace of mind. We need to lift the weight off our hearts and the crushing burdens off our shoulders that lead to heart issues, chest pain, neck pain and back pain. I'm becoming convinced that all this dis-ease and emotional pain ultimately turns into physical health problems, illness and cancer.

LIFE LESSON: LEARN TO RELAX

Make it a priority to enjoy life more. Become aware of the way you cope with pressure and stress and the effects they have on your mind and body. Practise some form of relaxation technique daily. Get help to do this if you need to such as group therapy, massage, hypnotherapy, acupuncture, yoga, joining a gym or a meditation class – whatever works for you.

1/1/2019 Tuesday

The palms of my hands and the soles of my feet are like frying pans they feel so hot. Had to get up at 11.30pm to take antacid – my oesophagus was on fire with indigestion. Must take that steroid tablet in the morning as soon as possible and the antihistamine tablet as well – the itchiness under my arms and all around the genital area wants to break out again. It's all about managing these awful side-effects. Have done my breast exercises to avoid contracting Lymphoma, due to having had the central lymph node removed during surgery – the cancer hadn't spread there, thank God! It was on the verge and just about to. Have been told by the oncology nurse I have to put skin moisturiser on hands and feet. Try not to have morning tea – the less I eat the better I feel. My hair has started to fall out in more obvious ways but I quickly tidy it up and put it in the bin. I don't want to be scared or depressed by it. My eyesight has been affected. I am reaching for John's reading glasses – never needed reading glasses before and my eyesight in general is blurry even with my glasses. It's okay though.

I know I've just got to get through this and then the body will start to heal again - this amazing body I'm beginning to have so much respect for.

As I sit in my comfortable chair and take some deep breaths, I say to myself: "Be strong – you can do it – you've got this! I can rely on you. You're a tough little cookie, and you are very loved. How lucky you are!"

2/1/2019 Wednesday

Trying to make sense of all this and unable to. Decide to read instead – I usually have a few books on the go at a time and at the moment I'm reading, *Harding's Luck* by E. Nesbit published in 1909 about a poor, 'lame' boy, as he is called in the story, who dreams of better things and discovers how to time travel into the past where he is healthy and rich and *Chronicles of Avonlea* by *Anne of Green Gables* author, L. M. Montgomery, also *Heal Your Body A–Z* by Louise L. Hay, *The Secret Language of Your Body* by Inna Segal and *The Hero with a Thousand Faces* by Joseph Campbell. I choose the Nesbit novel for this moment as I feel I need to do a bit of escaping right now. After reading a couple of chapters I do as much around the house as I can while I'm feeling okay.

3/1/2019 Thursday

Today there has been a big change in my hair. I've been losing a lot of it: quite a bit on my pillow in the morning, piles on my brush and I'm hardly touching it and heaps falling out like flakes of snow on my face, day and night. It's just falling out on its own. I can't wait to wash it tomorrow – can't wait another day – four days already since the last wash. I'm trying to wait as long as I can. I know one week is the ideal and has been recommended by the hospital but it's so hot and my head has been full of perspiration each day. Overall I feel pretty good – almost but not really my usual self. Stomach and food and drink still need special attention and I tend to lose my voice. Eyesight is weaker too, but still I feel better and much better than the first week of Chemo which is like a past nightmare that looms in the background.

4/1/2019 Friday

Clumps of my hair are falling out. It's scary. So much has fallen out that I fear there'll be nothing left, but I've braced myself for it. It's almost unbelievable, filling up the plug hole in the shower like a huge hairy hamster is blocking the drain, and still falling as I give it the gentlest of washes with the toxin free shampoo the oncology nurses have recommended - which is ironic considering the enormous quantities of toxins that have been pumped into me. When I get out and pat my hair dry, I notice that big lumps have matted like dreadlocks on top but most of those fall out too in big masses. This is horrible especially because it's happening so quickly and copiously. It's scary! Hopefully it will grow back. What a strange thing this is – so harsh and cruel – it's death! But ironically it means life. It's survival and if I can be strong enough, I will survive this and be stronger for it. I hate it in the meantime though, but I won't let it shake me too much. I know I am still me no matter what I look like.

I'm having a blood test this morning to make sure I can manage the next Chemo treatment and confirm that my body has sufficiently recovered to withstand the next assault. I admit I am scared about the next treatment – dreading it really – since I almost didn't get through that week after the first session. I'm relying on positive affirmations, so when the anxiety creeps in I try to push it aside with the most positive statements I can think of. It doesn't matter if I'm not fully convinced, I say them to myself anyway: "I am strong. I will be strong. I am stronger than I know. I have the courage of a lion. All is well."

I've found I can't have sweet snacks anymore. At the moment I'm amazed that I need substantial food – protein – meat and eggs and fish. I've never been much of a meat eater at all, especially since John's first triple heart bypass operation nearly thirty years ago and then the second – a quadruple one in 2007 we've both focussed on fruit and vegetables with fish and a little meat occasionally. But I have to put that aside right now. I need to have it, otherwise I feel hollow with a gnawing, empty feeling in my stomach. Right now my food needs to be plain, whole and solid and a little bit goes a long way but it has to be at least four or five small meals a day with plenty of vegetables, and cordial is enough of a drink – Golden Circle Apple and Raspberry.

It's very strange for me to be on this side of things: me the sick one having to think about each item of food and very careful about the way it's cooked; having to think about my every movement, my every task, making sure not to waste even an ounce of energy with people needing to look out for me and help me. I've always been the carer and I'm happy to help and to be helpful. I'm good at that – I'm not so good at thinking about what I need or want – that has always come last or not at all in my thinking. Now I'm forced to think about my own needs just to get through the day. Everything is turning out the opposite of what I've done before and I know I need to listen and learn. What I've done before has been too lopsided. I have never placed myself first in my own life. That's a silly thing to do – taking on other people's problems, hurts, worries and burdens. But it's no one else's fault – I've allowed that – I've been encouraged to do that throughout all my growing up years. I think it's like that for many women – family, society and religion all taught us that nothing about ourselves or our needs and wants was or ever would be as important as our partners, our children, our loved ones, all who came under our care and even strangers who happened to cross our path.

I can see it's time to make a change now. I've been forced to! Whatever it meant before and why, doesn't really count; it means this now: I have to focus on taking care of myself if I want to get through this.

Negative emotions such as anger, resentment, guilt, grief, rage, fear, unforgiveness, over a long time can turn into chronic illness. But it's not so simple – not all women who experience these things get breast cancer. I think it's part of the answer but nothing is ever the whole story as in Leonard Cohen's insightful *Anthem* song: "You can add up the parts but you won't have the sum." It's part of the answer but how many other millions of things have contributed and ultimately what does it matter? I can't really get to the bottom of it completely but I know one very definite fact: this disease and the treatment that follows it have forced me to live very much in the moment, more than ever before. The side-effects are so many and things can change so quickly in how I'm feeling that I'm grateful for each hour that is manageable and that I'm feeling pretty good. I'm grateful that I can enjoy a short walk and have some food that I like and spend quiet time reading or talking with John or my brother and sister and friends. I'm grateful that I don't feel nauseous and that all my limbs don't ache. I'm grateful that it's a cool day and not 42.8 degrees Celsius like yesterday was. And I'm grateful that I can wash and feed myself and go to the toilet and get myself a drink which was something my Mum couldn't do on her own for the last eight years of her life. I'm grateful I'm not in constant pain as she was and I'm grateful I have a loving, considerate husband when she had already been a widow for over six years. I'm grateful for my beautiful family and friends both close by and further away and I cherish each one of them. I'm grateful for the exceptional team of medical experts who are looking after me. In this moment I'm happy reviewing all the people and things I'm grateful for and I'm feeling okay and I know I'm very, very lucky.

LIFE LESSON: LIVE IN GRATITUDE

Make a list of everything you are grateful for in your life, including people, circumstances and things. When you feel low, review this list or just think about one of these points and then add one more thing to the list – it can be the smallest thing. The more you experience feelings of gratitude, the more you find to be grateful for - and the more you realise that life is one huge gift.

6/1/2019 Sunday Early Morning

Only one day before my next treatment and everything has settled down – my hands and feet aren't as hot; the itchiness has mostly subsided and I feel almost like a healthy person. The sunrise through the Silky Oaks in our back yard looks superb - glowing an apricot-pink. The birds are chirping and the garden looks green and peaceful. I can see the lorikeets on the branches puffing themselves up and doing their morning preening and washing. What a beautiful world it is!

6/1/2019 Late Afternoon

My second Chemo session tomorrow! I have to be at the hospital at 7.45 am to get ready for the treatment which begins at eight o'clock. I'm glad it's early so I don't need to wait around all day for it to happen. I can't wait for it and I dread it at the same time. I want to get it over and done with, then I'll be half-way through the treatment and that's a big achievement. At the very back of my mind, dread is looming like a crouching panther in the darkness but I won't let it pounce. I keep pushing aside any terrifying thought that tries to creep in and replacing it with a positive one. Hopefully all will be well and smooth – nothing like last time, but I can't help feeling a little bit scared of my reactions – no more of those, I hope, all smooth sailing and getting to the end without a hitch this time.

7/1/2019 Monday 5.05am

I have realised that lately I can't stop thinking about food. I've been eating like a horse and if it was in front of me I'd probably eat the actual horse. It's very strange as meat is not a food I've ever been attracted to or particularly wanted but right now it's the only thing that makes me feel full – meat, fish and maybe eggs. It seems I crave protein at the moment. Chocolate and sugary snacks don't interest me at all and as a sweets and chocolate lover it seems odd, but it could be the Dexmethsone I am taking each day to keep all the side effects under control – it's a steroid tablet and it works, but of course it has side effects too. I think my aversion to sweets might also be caused by the Chemo drugs themselves. Wherever it's coming from I can't ignore it. I've decided that this whole process of my treatment has to be the focus at the moment and it demands certain things if I want to get through it in the best way.

It's like a storm. You need to take shelter and do what you have to do to survive. I need to look after myself and do what I have to do with as much dignity as I can. I can't be prissy about this or wimpy. The foods I don't usually eat and the way I normally eat has to be put aside for now – even drinks etc. in fact everything about my life. It's only temporary and maybe I'll discover a new and better way by the end of this that gives me an even better, healthier life. This storm has to be weathered and I have to be strong and this food is helping to do that. Bless all the animals that are helping to see me through. I bless all of them with gratitude in my heart.

7.00pm

I have made it through a second Chemo treatment! I feel relieved but my head and eyes feel very heavy and my body feels very lethargic. It feels like I've been heavily sedated but I am managing and it's so much better than last time. There were no instant reactions or jolts or crazy symptoms today, so being at home is a blessing and I love it.

I'm back to not liking food or wanting any. The last few days I've been eating like a body builder so it's probably just as well. The little soup Maria made for me was enough – nutritious and brothy – perfect. A feeling of indigestion is creeping up even after such a little bit of food – must take antacid. The entire treatment really is a huge assault on the body with tablets, needles, wet hair plastered with conditioner, hard freezing cap on the head, drip and drugs into the back of the hand, sitting for four to five hours to get everything into the system. But the nurses make up for so much. Mel was so competent and nice. She explained everything about the new drug they replaced the Docetaxel with – all the side effects etc. It's more prone to cause heart problems but it's still the better choice for me. My hair has come out the worst from this – it is falling out constantly. The nurse said the cold cap doesn't work on everyone. Oh well! I've still got some hair left – just enough to look all right from a distance, but I've lost about half of it now.

8/1/2019 Tuesday

I feel unbalanced and dizzy but thankful that the second treatment is over and nothing drastic happened. I am at home and I feel okay – trying to do the waterfall meditation and turning it into a prayer. I do feel supported by the Angels and by God – The Divine – Love – Life – The Source – Our Life Force – all interchangeable terms. What a team I have surrounding me. There are so many helpers and I'm grateful to them all.

In the meantime, I'm becoming more and more bald – actually, balder and balder, despite the terrible discomfort of the cold cap – but it's okay; at least I've still got some hair left and that's something I suppose.

What's important in all this is to try to remain peaceful and not let the annoying small things take over and wreak havoc in my mind. When worries begin to rear their ugly heads, I need to do something else – don't give them free reign – get out of bed no matter what time it is – or go to another room and read or go outside and pull out a few weeds or phone a friend or do some cooking. Change the path I take – don't go down those familiar, unhappy tracks full of stress and anxiety that get me nowhere except feeling more pressured and tense. It makes no difference to anyone else – they are unaware of the tension I'm going through on their behalf. And as it's eating holes in my health, they are still doing whatever they want to do, while I'm going under.

Feeling constipated this morning but still went. Faeces is almost black and urine is reddish due to change in Chemo drug, but I'm glad I've been to the toilet – it gets rid of some of the toxins at least and it's a start. Feeling a bit nauseous too and don't care for any food. Feel generally okay though, thank God! So much hair falling of its own accord – hard to keep everything tidy with the flurry of hair. I'm listening to *The Lord of the Rings* tape by R.R. Tolkien and have begun reading the book again – for the third time – both times nearly half way through – this time I'd like to finish it – it's a fantastic story. I knew there was going to be the right time for me to read it – I've never half read any book in my life before and I've read thousands of them – so, it seems the worst time of my life is the perfect time for the best story.

9/1/2019 Wednesday 4am

Feeling very nauseous this morning – have taken tablet. Sucking on butterscotch lollies but they don't taste right. Reading *Lord of the Rings* and trying to focus on it instead. Will do meditations next.

10.30am

Feeling very low today – headachy, nauseous, dry cough, drained, heavy, dazed, constipated, retaining fluid, puffy in the face, losing plenty of hair. The shower drain is becoming blocked – John is trying to fix it. I gather all the hair I can but there's so much of it, I suppose some slips through down the plug hole. My feet and hands are back to being very hot and I'm generally feeling no good. All food tastes bad. The inside of my mouth tastes bitter like I've swallowed poison. My eyes feel tired and my eyelids are heavy. Have hardly any energy. Hopefully all will improve soon. I'm going to tick off yesterday right now and usher in a new, better time. My heart seems to beat harder too. But I will not focus on any of this – I just simply note that these symptoms and feelings are there and give myself that acknowledgement so I don't dismiss any of it – after all it is horrible and I am going through it and my body is taking a huge battering so there's no sense in pretending, but now it's time to move on from that. I've ticked off eight days already from this month – a huge achievement! I feel more hopeful already.

4.00pm

Had a small walk around the backyard. I feel weak: headachy and heavy, slow and old, unsteady on my feet, not able to focus properly, my eyes are a bit blurry – frail and feeble, that's how I feel, but still a bit better than this morning. Started to improve slightly around 2.30pm. I feel very numb but it's better than earlier so I'm grateful and hoping that tomorrow brings a better day health-wise.

10/1/2019 Thursday

Made it through the night without having to get up for hours in the middle. I don't feel that I've slept at all but I think I must have been very lightly dozing. I don't care. I got through it and it's morning and I can tick another day off as soon as I've spoken to Vincent. I have completed twenty-four days of Chemo – 24 days closer to the end of it! Yesterday my body didn't feel my own. It puffed up and was bloated. I looked different. I asked John and he agreed with what I was saying – very tentatively – he didn't want to hurt my feelings but it was obvious that I didn't look right. I didn't look like me at all and I was very unsteady on my feet and off balance. Throughout the night my mouth had a horrible, strange taste in it and now my stomach is starting to feel bad again. I don't know if it's better to have something to eat or not to. I don't want anything but maybe it will help if I do. I want to help myself as much as possible to have a good day.

One thing I have discovered about all of this is I can get up anytime I want to and it's all right. John goes back to sleep. I don't have to be apologetic about it and feel that I have disturbed him too much. He is working hard and I don't want to interrupt his sleep. Both of us have always worked hard. I know all work must bring some pressure and I'm more aware of that than ever. I want to let up on all of it and from now on choose, choose, choose to do only the things I love to do or at the very least want to do and not do things anymore under a sense of obligation or the feeling that I should or must do it. I need to be free in my body, my mind and my actions – in everything - so that I can begin to enjoy life much, much more while there's still some time left.

I have put stupid restrictions on myself – unnecessary restrictions that made no difference to anyone else but have restricted my own life – such as not doing things I might have enjoyed because I didn't think it was important enough if it was only for me. I think when you always put yourself last, it's not a good thing. In the past I have mixed up looking after yourself with selfishness. It's not selfish to put yourself first in your own life – that's how it should be. Then you can have others beside you and take good equal care of them instead of depleting yourself at every turn and trying to keep going when you haven't got much energy left. If you do this over a long time you leave the way open for resentment to creep in and spoil any good thing you might have done. And it's no one's fault but your own because you haven't managed to find the balance in your life.

Have a runny nose. Couldn't swallow the toast and it had no taste – when toast isn't good, well, nothing much more needs to be said. I had to spit it out – it was too dry and wouldn't go down even with the margarine.

I'm having some peeled, raw ginger in boiling water as a way of something to drink that might settle my stomach. I've found a word that sums up this Chemo as far as I can think right now – it's "dreadful" – absolutely <u>dreadful</u>. It is an assault on your whole being, on your entire body, mind and spirit. I feel like a small, hunted animal, trying to stay alive, looking furtively around me – not even sure what I'm watching out for – now I remember – the Dexmethsone's side effect is anxiety and it really does kick in fairly quickly. I've felt quite silly a couple of times when the tears set in, until I suddenly remembered again that it's the tablet. My memory has been affected too by these treatments. I think I can truthfully say every particle of me has been affected. The Dexmethsone itself is to combat the symptoms and side-effects of the two big Chemo drugs, so it's necessary and helpful – everything has to be managed and balanced – ironic as I have never felt so out of balance. Hold strong! Hold strong, girl, you can do it! You know you have hidden strengths in you yet to be revealed. You are stronger than even you know! Look what has come at you in the past and you got through it all and helped others as well. This is not much different; it's just another experience to get through, to learn from, to take the blessing out of and to discard the rest forever. So, what's the blessing? There may be more than one. A bit more patience is needed and endurance. You can do it! Draw on what you've done before and accept help – human, divine, animal, mineral and vegetable – all the help that comes your way and be grateful <u>*not*</u> apologetic about it.

8.40pm

What a hard, harsh day!

Had to go into hospital to have an enema I was so blocked up and in pain. Tried to go to the toilet for ten hours – since 5.00am this morning and felt like I badly needed to go but couldn't go. It got worse as the day went on – couldn't sit, stand or do anything and feeling more blocked in both faeces and urine. I tried absolutely everything including suppositories which John went to the chemist to buy. I'd been given some numbers by the oncology nurses to call in case I needed advice or help but I didn't want to do that if I could help it. I eventually realised there was nothing else I could do and I was in a lot of pain. The day oncology nurse told me to go into the emergency department at the hospital when I phoned to ask her about it. She said to go straight away but I tried for another half an hour to no avail. I feel exhausted and weary now but so glad we went because it couldn't unblock by itself. It all seemed to get out of hand so quickly till I was in real distress and unable to cope with it while it worsened by the hour.

It was a long, stressful, uncomfortable and hard-fought day full of suffering. The relief I feel is immense as is the gratitude I feel to all those who helped me.

11/1/2019 Friday 5.10am

After a horrendous day – one of my very worst, I got through the night with only one toilet break. I feel a bit nauseous now with a strange, sickly-sweet taste in my mouth. I had to get up. Had Weeties and anti-nausea tablet, ginger in hot water and hope for the best. I am puffy and bloated. I don't look like myself at all. I feel all misshapen. This new Chemo drug is causing this puffiness, nausea, bloating and bad constipation – but it doesn't matter – I have to remind myself that I will come back as well as I can, as good as I can, and as strong as I can. This will pass and I will be better, and I can tick off another day done!

I'm finding there is always hope – something positive – even a tiny thing that gives me the little boost I need to keep going because there were moments yesterday when I was weary, depressed, desperate and in terrible pain in my entire gut and genital areas – so much so that I thought, "What is this all for? There is no dignity in any of this – just pain and suffering." The doctors and nurses were lovely, of course! They were careful, understanding and very competent. I couldn't have asked for better care – it was just something that had to be done. I hadn't realised things could get out of hand so quickly. I keep forgetting my body is not normal at the moment and what might have been a simple thing before the Chemo can quickly turn into an alarming if not life-threatening episode. I felt like saying, "Enough! I've had enough of all this! I can't do it anymore!"

But today I've had Weeties and my anti-nausea tablet and maybe I can inch my way through another day closer to the end of this treatment. I'm thinking that surely with all the amazing geniuses and brains in this world there could be a better cure than this. Instead of working to destroy each other, if the focus of the human race could be on health and healing, we'd all be in heaven on earth. I sometimes think that maybe what these strong, crazy people need is a serious bout of illness or disease to wake them up to their own mortality because if they were thinking straight, surely they wouldn't behave in the destructive way they do – that goes from some world leaders to everyday aggressive troublemakers.

12/1/2019 Saturday 3.30am

I'm immersed in *Lord of the Rings* with Frodo pursued by the "Black Riders" and he's running from peril into more peril. I feel too wide awake to sleep. I'm trying to feel peaceful – am enjoying the book very much and this time will read it through to the end. Not sure about anything else right now except that I'd love to get another three to four hours of sleep. I hope it happens but how do I get myself sleepy enough?

I have to use John's reading glasses to read now – my eyesight is weaker since this treatment. I'm hoping it will all be restored – can it be at sixty? Who knows? I suppose I'm lucky to be able to read at all or to be alive at this age.

I trust and I will continue to trust that I am being looked after by all the Divine good and all the good people around me who have been helping me get through with their help and prayers and their genuine concern and support. God bless them all. I gratefully receive all the help I can get. I need every little bit of it.

LIFE LESSON: ACCEPT HELP

Ask for help when you need it. Be open to all the love and the good that comes to you and accept it graciously. Try to get out of the mindset that you have to be the giving one all the time. It means a lot to those who love you to know they have been able to help you in some way. Giving and receiving have to be in healthy balance in your life.

4.00am

Back in bed again. My body is raging with all the chemicals in it – just hot as hell – my feet are frying, my hands are hot, my head is aching, my stomach is in revolt, my face and eyes are puffy – every part of me is feeling wrong.

6.20am

Up and ready for the day. Have a very runny nose, terrible taste in my mouth. After eating anything there's a bitter taste left behind; feel nauseous. Have taken anti-nausea tablet – ready to take Dexmethsone now. Having ginger in hot water – hoping all this settles down right now.

<u>27 Days Done</u>

13/1/2019 Sunday 2.00am

I feel so sick in the stomach. I need to take an anti-nausea tablet now. I have to eat something or I feel I still will vomit – biscuits, shortbread, crystalised ginger – I don't want any of it but I have to have something – a Salada biscuit, a butterscotch lolly. I'm having everything I can to stave off this horrible queasiness. Salt mouthwash next and a cup of hot water after that – this is horrible. Now I won't be able to go to bed till I can digest all this. I thought I might feel better today but this is not a good start.

In "Lord of the Rings", I follow Frodo on his long, slow, perilous journey through the Old Forest. He feels he's going from one danger into the next when suddenly he finds himself alone and crying miserably for his friends who are somewhere behind him. He's frightened and so am I – this is only the first part of a long and treacherous journey, set with pitfalls and traps. No matter how much I do everything the medical staff say to keep me on track, these "medicines" are playing hell with my body – my dear, enduring, fighting, brave, little body. I'll try and help it as much as I can.

10am.

Got a little bit of sleep after I went back to bed but I feel very quivery and shaky today and very numb – everywhere I touch on my body, especially around my face and head. I'm disappointed too – I thought I'd feel better than this, but I feel very weak and sick instead.

14/1/2019 Monday 6.30am

Had a much better night. Slept 3-4 hours but didn't have to get up – rested and prayed. This morning I have woken up feeling better. Have had breakfast to try to get the dreadful taste out of my mouth. Had Weeties, porridge, one piece of toast (grain bread) a slice of green apple, 4 cherries, 4 blueberries, 2 slices of banana, ginger in hot water. I feel very weak in the legs and knees and very quivery inside the stomach and all over. Hoping it passes soon. Now the magpies are calling me – it's Josephine and her baby. Since Josephine broke her leg and John and I helped her through it, she comes more often, bringing her husband, Napoleon, and her two babies. We always greet them with warmth and welcome and so they've become part of our family.

7.40am

This ever-changing condition is very hard to handle: I've had to take an anti-nausea tablet and don't feel good at all right now. Went to the toilet though and I'm relieved that food is working its way through and not blocking like a stone.

2.20pm

I truly didn't know I had been in such danger till one and a half hours ago when I spoke to my surgeon, Julia. She told me plainly that the cancer I had was a very fast-growing one and wouldn't respond to the usual oestrogen medications. It was Triple Negative – which I already knew and much more aggressive than I had realised. I now realise, finally, that I came very close to it not being caught and contained at all. It was at the last stage of Stage One where it was about to pounce and start spreading. My next mammogram wasn't due for another year. That happy 'chance' of the discharge from my right breast that happened last year was what alerted our family doctor of over thirty-five years, Doctor Frankel, that there was trouble. He immediately sent me off on a course of exploratory tests which detected the hidden enemy lurking and aggressively spreading quickly in my right breast. I can hardly believe it but as I tell my brother and sister, it seems they were already aware of the danger and the seriousness of it. It was only I who all along thought it was unreal and down-played it as though it was nothing. When I first saw Julia, I asked, "Are you sure it's not a mistake?" "There's no mistake," she had replied, calmly but firmly. I still didn't believe. I thought there must be a mix up. I was never ill – certainly not with anything serious and I didn't feel ill now. It just didn't make sense so I wasn't going to focus on it. Consequently, I went into the initial tests and surgery with a sense of unreality and fearlessness. I think that may have been for the best.

Today when I was at a very low ebb and struggling so much with all the side-effects of the Chemo, I wanted to ask again if it was all necessary. Julia was very understanding, calm and compassionate. She said plainly that it's a balancing act between the benefits and the side-effects of all the drugs and that it was my choice. In the conversation I remembered to ask what sort of cancer I had and it was then that she fully enlightened me. I think she may have done last time I saw her as well but that time I didn't hear it. I probably wasn't ready. I wasn't interested in any of the details. I took in only what I needed to know to get me through.

This time I heard it loud and clear and now I understand why I have to go through this and why everything has to be done to prevent it coming back again and why I am so lucky for it to have been caught just in time before it destroyed me. It's miraculous! I find it hard to believe. I am so lucky. John understood all along. He is not hearing anything new. But I've heard it now and it gives me new vigour and new strength to keep going and feel glad that I have been given a second chance at life. Now I know how fortunate I've been and I won't waste the opportunity to get to the other side of this horrible thing that has crept in to destroy my life. I have to make sure it is totally gone and to remove all patterns of thought and behaviour which may have contributed, caused or encouraged it. I am on the alert now. I am fully aware. My eyes have been opened and I'm ready to step forward into a new, brighter, healthier, happier life.

LIFE LESSON: RELY ON THE EXPERTS

Be aware of the treatment you are undergoing, ask questions and make decisions, but ultimately you have to trust that the doctors looking after you are working in your best interest. Once you have assured yourself that you have a great team of medical experts, listen to them, trust them and follow their advice. They know a lot more about the treatment of this condition than you do. If you fight them and stand in their way you are standing in your own way of getting better.

15/1/2019 Tuesday 5.14am

I'm so happy that it's morning already and I can get up. I've made it through the night with quite good sleep and I feel not too bad this morning. I have a new resolve today of getting through all this in the best way I can, knowing I'm on the right track for me and not having to second guess myself every moment. Up till now I've continually questioned whether having Chemo was completely necessary for me. What a lot of wasted energy! After the specialist visit yesterday and speaking to Julia, I finally realised I need to do this one hundred per cent – not because she said I should but because I finally understood the severity of what I've had and the danger I was in.

The taste in my mouth is terrible. My stomach was on fire yesterday. Had antacid at the end but it still scares me that something could block me up like last time and I want to avoid that almost more than anything else. I'm going to be extremely careful about everything I eat and drink today.

I'm already half-way through this month. Congratulations and celebrations! While I want to get through these treatments as soon as possible, I don't want to wish my life away. In this dire circumstance, I think the best I can do is live in the present moment and enjoy any contact I have with family and friends as I can clearly feel their genuine love and concern for me. I love them all so much and am so grateful for their presence in my life. When Frodo finally learns who is pursuing him and why, he says faintly, "Thank goodness I did not realise the horrible danger....I was mortally afraid, of course, but if I had known more, I should not have dared even to move. It is a marvel that I escaped!"

I am just reading this today. It seems to run parallel to my thoughts and is very insightful and strange. Yes, I agree – I had no idea of the danger that was averted when I had breast surgery to remove the two malignant tumours – one 16mm across. All I can think is: "Thank goodness I escaped." I didn't even know I was in any real danger, and perhaps it was better that way. I just kept going forward in a hazy, is this real? sort of way.

1.15pm

My new resolve is to completely remove the word, "should" from my vocabulary. No more obligation as the incentive – do things because I want to, I choose to, I love to do them.

16/1/2019 Wednesday 1.20pm

A terrible numbness has descended on me – even my teeth are numb – my head especially. I feel so out of it. I feel dreadful. The numbness has never left me since this second treatment but today it is worse rather than better. I don't know why – maybe because I only had two and a half hours sleep last night but now we have just had lunch so I can't lie down for a long while or I'll get terrible indigestion as I've discovered the hard way from past experience. This is horrible right now. I pray that it passes quickly.

I keep thinking I can do more to help myself get better quicker and try and help with the housework and I hadn't realised I was putting so much pressure on myself until I spoke to my sister this morning on the phone. Maria said to me in her usual straight forward and funny way, "Sis, remember you're as sick as you can get before being nailed in! You need to look after yourself more." I have always placed many expectations on myself, punished myself in subtle ways and spoken to myself in harsh words. I'm starting to see that this is the pattern of a lifetime for me – a pattern that needs to be changed – that I need to change!

17/1/2019 Thursday

This is my best morning so far in this second treatment. I feel almost myself and I've slept for five to six hours. This is a great beginning to a new day. I look forward to better times ahead in every way.

1.25pm

I see how things can change in extreme ways very quickly from hour to hour during this process. It surprises and at times scares me. From feeling quite reasonable earlier, now I feel done in. My energy is so very low and the taste in my mouth is bitter and terrible. It seems that this second Chemo treatment is terrible in different ways. My heart keeps beating fast and hard at times all of its own accord as though I've been running, when I'm just sitting in a chair with hardly energy enough to move. And the horrible taste in my mouth – and nothing can change it – except liquorice. My sister gave me a long, curled up liquorice strap and I can actually taste it. I'm stunned and happy. My stomach still plays havoc and is ready to wreak a wild fire at every turn.

18/1/2019 Friday

Have had a chest problem that is slowly getting worse - wheezing badly at night and unable to sleep. Have been put immediately on antibiotics by Emma, my oncologist. I had to phone her this morning about the chest and she sent a prescription through to the local chemist, saving me a trip into the hospital – just as well as I feel shocking and have almost zero energy.

19/1/19 Saturday

Chest wheezing is still bad. For the first time I have given in to feeling sorry for myself. Stupidly have been crying about having to deal with this extra thing. It just seemed to overwhelm me for a while. Then I spoke to Vincent and felt a lot better. I felt a bit of improvement this afternoon and happily ticked another day off the calendar. I've been doing that after my phone call with Vincent each day which is something I look forward to. I know it's not easy for him as he and his wife, Lorrie have their own serious health issues but right now it helps me a lot to get that phone call and to know they care about what's happening with me even if they are in Queensland. I know I'm getting lots of help through family and friends who are praying for me and constantly sending me good wishes through emails and texts and respecting the fact that I haven't got the energy to see people at the moment or to talk much on the phone.

20/1/2019 Sunday 5.10am

Have well and truly stopped feeling sorry for myself – what a waste of effort it all was anyway! Feeling better this morning – not as much wheezing if I don't talk. Have taken antibiotic tablet immediately and am starting to get over this chest congestion/infection too. What a marvellous body it is to be so resilient and fight on!

21/1/2019 Monday 5.10am

Still wheezy in the chest but not as bad as yesterday. Will have to go to the doctor tomorrow. Every little thing seems to turn into something huge and can quickly get out of hand. It shows I have to be extra careful and act on any symptoms or side-effects without delay.

22/1/2019 Tuesday

One thing I have learnt out of this is to live in the

moment – enjoy the present, enjoy this moment. It saves so much worrying and fretting – worrying about what you should've, could've, would've done in the past if only you had known this or that or realised before you said or did that and stressing about what may happen in the future that may never happen at all. And worrying and fretting on behalf of other people and their lives, when they are often perfectly okay with how things are going for them, but we feel they could be doing such a lot better if only they would listen to us. Let go! Let go! Let go! And focus on your own life, your own happiness, your own relaxation and on how to make things better for you and then those around you will get the benefit of all that release of tension and feel happier and more relaxed themselves and if you really need to say something, say it once – you've done your job – then let it make a difference or not make a difference – it's up to that person to decide if they will listen, act on it or pay any attention at all; it's not up to you. Stop trying to control, twist, manipulate outcomes in other people's lives — even with the best intentions – it's enough if you can make your own life work. Can people look at you and say: "Now that's an example of real happiness!" otherwise stop trying to fix things. Focus on your own life and getting it right – the rest is often an excuse for not wanting to deal with your own problems or not wanting to admit there are any. And another major thing this extreme experience has confirmed for me is to treat people with as much love as you can and be generous in every way you can be. I've found these are the things I look back on with regret – the instances when I wasn't loving enough or generous in my dealings with others.

23/1/2019 Wednesday 4.35am

Very hard to sleep during the night so I have decided to get up and take my first antibiotic tablet for the day and pretend it's not all that early. I've been really disturbed by the fact that my sister has caught this infection from me. I thought it was something to do with Chemo so I wasn't even careful, coughing and spluttering all over the place and now she might have this horrible chest thing. I'm just hoping it will have already lifted off by the morning.

Yesterday when I went to see our G.P. Doctor Frankel, he quickly put a mask on and put one on me. As it turned out, what I have is something infectious and I thought it was just because I am in a weak state. It *is* in an indirect way but I'm really annoyed with myself for not being more careful around Maria and John and not realising that it was something catchy. The truth is too that I'm sick of all this: I'm sick of being careful and sick of being sick, and sick of doctors and hospitals and needles and not feeling well.

24/1/2019 Thursday 3.30am

Finding it hard to sleep, otherwise I'm feeling quite a bit better now. It's only three days to the next Chemo treatment and this chest infection needs to clear up completely – this has been an extra complication I really didn't need.

25/1/2019 Friday 5.48am

The weather has been so hot. It was 30 degrees overnight with a predicted 43 degrees today. I've already been up nearly an hour, taken cough medicine and my antibiotic tablet which needs to be taken half an hour before food three times a day. Today we have to go to the doctor's clinic to find out about the chest x-ray results he sent me to have done. I was hoping we could save ourselves the trip in this heat but I wasn't able to get any results over the phone.

I am feeling better today but I still have a cough and I'm still wheezing a bit in the chest. The x-rays have shown that I have bronchitis. I have to have a blood test today because of the next Chemo treatment on Tuesday. It's a merry-go-round and it seems at the moment there's no getting off. I have to go with it and try to be okay with it all when I'm not really okay with any of it.

27/1/2019 Sunday 5.57am

Couldn't sleep. Got up at 3.00am for an hour. John got up too. We watched a bit of an old movie – lately we've been watching some 1930s films we've never seen before. They've been showing in the early hours of the morning – "The Falcon in Mexico," in Hollywood, in San Francisco etc. and "The Saint in New York," in Palm Springs, in London etc.- between the Falcon and the Saint we've done a lot of travelling on our couch in the eighteen movies so far.

Now I'm up for the day. My chest is still wheezing a bit. Took my antibiotic tablet. I hope today to be totally well and the bronchitis gone as well as the chest congestion. What a struggle it's been in the last two weeks over this. I hate being sick. I'm scared about the next Chemo treatment. The drugs have such a terrible effect. My balance was so bad after the last treatment that I could hardly stand or walk to the car without falling. I only vaguely remember clinging to John's arm.

We are seeing the specialist before the treatment this time. Dear God, I hope it's still the same number of treatments and no more due to these complications. I can hardly cope with these. I've had a bad headache the last couple of days. I'm thinking it could be caused by the heat or maybe it's the infection or the Chemo I've already had. Who knows? And my neck hurts terribly. Twice this week I've had to go in to the hospital for x-rays. Each week so far has presented new problems. I hope this next treatment is easy in every way because I don't have much energy. I've lost about half my hair. It's not nice but I can cope with that. It's all these other things that crop up that I'm finding hard to handle because they come on top of all the Chemo side-effects. I know they are indirectly caused by the Chemo which has compromised my immune system. Now every little thing blows up out of all proportion and quickly becomes a serious health issue. I know it's different for everyone, as the oncology nurses have told me, but for me, the Chemotherapy has been really horrendous and that's just simply the truth without embellishment or exaggeration.

28/1/2019 Monday 5.35am

I had a really good night's sleep – the soundest in over two weeks at least – only got up once during the night. This is the day before the next Chemo treatment and it remains to be seen if I'm well enough to have it. I never want to have another one again but if I have to – and I know I do – then I want to get it over and done with as soon as possible, so I hope I'm well enough.

I've heard it said that if you look at your life in the present moment you can see what your past beliefs have created. If that's true then it means I haven't loved myself enough and any major health problems may be rooted in self-neglect. I'm suffering, I'm going to have more pain inflicted on my body and I still have a long way to go before I have finished all these treatments. I haven't ever really paid attention to what I wanted or needed. I didn't think it was important. My role - or so I have thought – has been to support others – my husband, my parents, my siblings and anyone else who has come into my sphere and has needed something – and that's most people I've ever met. This is obvious stuff – it's not a bad thing to help others – of course not! – it's the best thing – it's only not so good when you help others to the exclusion of yourself – when you push yourself into the background till you hardly exist – and when that becomes the pattern of your life then you don't really have a life. And when you don't really have a life maybe your body says, "Well then, I'm out of here!" I'm not certain about this but that's how it seems at the moment.

I do know we give away our freedom and power so quickly and easily to those around us, especially in our late teens and early twenties when we're forming partnerships. So much hurt and abuse of power happens because often we don't see or realise what we're allowing – what patterns we're setting up, what permission we're giving as to how we will be treated, what boundaries and lack of boundaries we're establishing, what rods we're making for our own backs that may last a lifetime. Why on earth would you ever want to clamp yourself into chains? Yet nearly all of us do at some point in our lives, making choices and decisions that lock us into situations which are difficult to get out of such as partnerships, marriages, businesses and promises we don't want to break, without knowing all the consequences.

One area that I've seen causing endless hurt in people's lives, including my own family is divorce. I think society has got this all wrong. I have been very blessed in my relationship with John which has lasted over forty years but many partnerships and marriages are not meant to last a lifetime. Those that do are uncommon – most are meant to last for a short time – sometimes weeks or months – some maybe a few years or a decade or two. If everyone could understand and accept this, instead of making people feel guilty and forcing them to stay together, how much of a happier place the world would be. I also believe there's an important purpose at the heart of every relationship, whether it is long term or a fleeting one and if the church and society would stop putting unreal pressure and expectations onto everyone and stop preaching, "it's the way God intended it" – which is a load of rubbish – people would be a lot healthier.

29/1/2019 Tuesday

Saw the specialist, my oncologist, Emma, this morning at 8.30am and she confirmed the Chemo treatment will go ahead at 12.30pm. My bronchitis is clearing and I'm feeling much better. I'm glad there won't be any delays. I want to keep ticking off the days and get closer to the end of this.

7.00pm

The discomfort is over. The session is finished. That horrible cold cap is off and I've got through another treatment. Had to go twice to the toilet while it was happening – a real nuisance because I had to roll in the drip stand and attachments and my head gear. My urine was red – quite unsettling - because of the Epirubicin drug. When I tell the nurse she is amazed that it is working through me so quickly, "but then it is administered intravenously," she says. "So, it has instant effect," I add in my own mind. Like last time, she waits by my side for fifteen minutes each time the two drugs are injected into the drip, to make sure there are no unexpected reactions. She tells me that if the drug backs up in the needle and blocks, it could flow out and burn my skin – but if that's one of the big concerns what's it doing when it actually goes into my body? Best not to think about it much.

I can see the tiny vials sitting on the tray in front of me – such little things – about one and a half inches tall and about an inch around but what's in them is so powerful and can have such dire consequences. I'm nervous and scared about it. I pray to be given the strength and courage to be brave and to be able to endure it without bad reactions.

I do endure it and we were home at 6.00pm. It's been a long day but all has been successful. Now if I can stave off the constipation, maybe I can handle these next three weeks better. I feel very dazed and dozy; it's because of the tablet under my tongue given to me just before the treatment, to help with the pain and discomfort of the cold cap. I didn't know this before. Half a tablet is suggested this time as John tells the nurse how unsteady on my feet I was for days last time and how I walked away from the treatment as though I was drunk. I can hardly remember. I don't feel quite as bad this time.

30/1/2019 Wednesday

I have to go to the local doctor's clinic for my white blood cells injection to be administered by the nurse although I have to see the doctor first. This has to happen each time after a Chemo session to help boost my white cells as the drugs kill off the good and bad blood cells alike. All has gone well and I'm glad it's over. I don't feel the heaviness and aching in the legs and the incredible fatigue in my body like I did the last two times when I could hardly drag myself around for a few feet at a time. I think my body is getting used to this assault on it. The body is a wondrous thing – wanting to heal itself and be well as fast as possible. I believe that all I need to do is work with it and I will be well.

31/1/2019 Thursday

I've been reminded by my body not to do things in a rush – I've got to slow everything down. Last night I had my two laxative tablets at once and it gave me indigestion even after taking the antacid to help with it. I still have indigestion this morning. It's as though my body is saying, "Take time for yourself; be gentle with yourself. Where are you rushing to get to? Don't let yourself feel a false sense of security just because you might be feeling a little better. Go carefully and monitor all the side-effects, that way avoiding them developing into something serious that requires going to the doctor or the hospital."

I've been up since 4.15am – now it's 6.45am. I've had breakfast: porridge, Weeties, one slice wholemeal toast, half a small tub blueberry yoghurt, small tub diced peaches in syrup, two glasses water – all to help with toilet – and it worked, so I have been successfully staving off the horrendous constipation following the second Chemo treatment which led to that emergency visit to the hospital.

This morning the burning sensation in my genital area has returned. I have taken an antihistamine tablet and at lunch I will take two more Dexmethsone tablets and hopefully bring it under control before it turns into that uncontrollable itchiness that is one of the worst things ever. Now I always put a rug down on any vinyl or leather chairs or couches to prevent perspiration when sitting down. One other stupid thing I did last night was to go to bed when I wasn't feeling sleepy. If I had stayed up for another hour I would probably have had a better night's sleep. I've found I'm better off staying up when I feel so sick.

My feet are starting to feel very hot again – I'll put moisturiser on them and on my hands the way I have been doing as per instruction guidelines. It's a full-time job just to get through all of this. I don't know how anyone can go to work or do anything else. Maybe they don't have the allergies and side-effects. The sixty-five-year-old man sitting next to me in the hospital was sipping a can of lemonade while he was having his Chemo treatment. I can't drink anything fizzy unless

I want horrible indigestion, and lemonade to me at the moment has the oddest taste that I honestly can't describe it's so weird and completely undrinkable – so we are all different. But his nails were turning a dark colour and the nurses were concerned and phoned his specialist. His wife pointed to my black-painted nails and I told them about how it's meant to help them stay on. The Chemo drugs can make the fingernails and toenails drop off and the black nail polish helps prevent that from happening by blocking out the light. I have been doing this since the first session as was suggested by the nurse. I find it hateful but if it helps me in any way then I'll do it. I remember in the past seeing women my age with black nail polish on short, stubby nails and thinking, "That looks hideous!" never realising in my ignorance that they were probably going through Chemo – and I thought I wasn't a judgemental person!

In the meantime, the big man next to me was fitted with cold gloves and didn't like it till his wife pointed out that I had a cold cap on my head for four and a half hours! So that stopped him complaining.

1/2/2019 Friday

Have finished reading the eight Narnia Chronicles, *The Lord of the Rings*, the Psamead Trilogy by E. Nesbit: *Five Children and It*, *The Phoenix and the Carpet* and *The Story of the Amulet* as well as *The Magic City* and have loved them all. I'm trying to make sure that each day apart from reading, I listen to music and do movements to it like dancing and even singing along and although I have hardly any voice left and I hardly have the energy to move, I really push myself to do these things as I've been told by my specialists that movement and activity speed up the healing process.

A lovely lady phoned me through an organisation at the hospital, trying to get me involved in a workshop about headscarves. She asked me how I was going and was I keeping up with walks and exercises and doing all the things suggested by the reading material I was given. I said I was. She had no idea how sick I felt and how it was hard for me to get from one side of the room to the other with all the pain and discomfort I had. She gave me some internet links and said I could look them up but I could tell she felt disappointed I wasn't doing more. How could I explain to her I couldn't do more? I was already forcing myself to move, to eat, to drink, when I didn't feel like doing any of those things and she couldn't understand because her strong, bouncy, enthusiastic voice through the phone told me that she was well, that she was fit and healthy and had plenty of energy and plenty to spare and I have practically none and that it was a big effort just to talk to her on the phone as I hardly have any voice and it's a struggle to make the words come out of my throat. "She has no idea how sick I am," I thought as I listened to her, "or what it means to feel this sick. That's okay it's not her fault."

I was as pleasant as possible and thanked her for her call. I knew she was well-meaning and well-intentioned and I'm sure the organisation helps many people – but not me. I need different things and I accept that most people don't realise that. Who can understand how sick I feel? Even those around me can't fully know how horrible this is. It's like trying to survive after having swallowed a bottle of poison that's wreaking havoc in my body and sapped almost every ounce of energy. Of course, I'm resolved to get through but why do some people expect you to pretend it's not as bad as it is? It's a hateful process and that's all that can be said about it. Just summon everything that's in you and make a resolution to get through and while you're at a low ebb, try to have as little to do with healthy, fit people as you can because many of them can't understand how weak and debilitated you feel.

I've felt very uncomfortable in the stomach today, flushed in the cheeks and horrible in the mouth, but I've got through. The day is nearly over and I can tick one more off. Lots to be grateful for – and it was cool weather today too – only 24 degrees in the middle of summer!

2/2/2019 Saturday 5.04am

I find I can read all the booklets and pamphlets on understanding Chemotherapy and related topics now. I couldn't look at them much before without feeling worse. They should include in the pamphlets: "Just be prepared to accept that you're going to be a human pin cushion!" with all the injections required. It's good to know I've been doing all the right things to help myself as much as I can. It's still hard though and frightening and I wonder if everything will come good again or at least come back, such as clear thinking, my sense of smell and taste, my energy, a nice thick head of hair as I've become bald on top and could easily join the Friars Minor without needing to shave the special patch. It would be so good if this sickly feeling in my stomach could be gone for good, the horrible taste in my mouth not be there anymore, and to be able to sleep through a night without needing to get up for a couple of hours. I know my life can't be the same after this – it's not meant to be. My hope is that it can be better, but physically I just don't know. I have an ulcer on the tip of my tongue. It appeared overnight and I don't know why as I've been doing my mouthwashes dutifully. I can only think I need more vegetables and soupy food so I will try that today.

3/2/2019 Sunday 5.08am

Have been awake for a couple of hours but I feel okay. I may as well be up as I can't sleep and that way John can probably snooze better and I can read. I can understand completely now why some people refuse to have treatment if their cancer has spread – it's because there isn't much hope of stopping it and most of all because the treatments take away all quality of life. You don't even feel like a human being most of the time – you just feel like a sick lump of yuckiness – you can't smell anything, you can't taste anything, your vision is fuzzier than usual, you feel dizzy, your brain doesn't function properly, you have no energy to do anything, your voice is gone so it's an effort to talk, you're not up to being around people. Nothing is enjoyable or fun. You have to push yourself to move due to so much fatigue, and force yourself to eat and drink in small mouthfuls and sips so you don't choke – it's very easy to choke as inside your throat feels swollen while your mouth tastes like you swallowed poison and your stomach feels horrible.

It truly is a test of survival – can I survive this treatment? I know that the whole area of cancer treatment is far better than it used to be and is improving all the time, but now in 2019 it is still terrible and something you would never wish anyone to go through unless there was absolutely no other way to save their life and even then, it must be their choice because this is a horrendous thing to have to go through. The choice has been much easier for me because the cancer hadn't spread – it was caught just in time but for those people who have gone beyond that stage and it has metastasised, I would never want to judge their decision.

It might sound dramatic to people who are well but without any exaggeration I feel that because of my allergy to the medication, this treatment has taken me to the brink of death – at moments, as close to it as I ever want to be and still be alive. Sometimes when my breath comes in an involuntary gasp or my heart starts palpitating unexpectedly when I'm just sitting in a chair, resting, it's frightening, and I know that while these drugs are hopefully helping me, they are also destroying me. My job is to find that balance, build myself up and get my way back to good health and to keep reminding myself constantly that I am one of the luckiest ones: my cancer has not spread and has been caught in time to save my life. It spurs me on to be positive and not allow the negativity to engulf me. I will work with the best that is available to me to make sure it doesn't return.

11.15am

I've been feeling very depleted today – no energy – very weak in the legs, no voice, a tremor throughout my body. We just went to my sister's for morning tea – no tea for me though – I have an aversion to all hot drinks, just a bit of cordial or water and I don't like the taste of either. Had one and a half scones Maria made; I can't appreciate their flavour but they look lovely and I can physically feel their fluffy consistency in my mouth. It has perked me up a little bit and I leave feeling I might need to go to the toilet. I do go as soon as I get home. The faeces is in the shape of a big stone just like when I got blocked up and had to go into emergency. It feels like my body is not my own. It's scary and shocking to think that has just come out of me but I feel better for having gone. I can see that if I'm not fully aware and remain vigilant about this, I could easily get blocked up again.

Now that I've eaten the scones and jam my mouth feels devoid of all saliva and my teeth are full of food sticking to them. I need to do a mouthwash right away to stop this sensation of dry teeth sticking to the inside of my mouth. Once I've done all that, I do feel better but very tired, as though I've done a full day's very hard work. I don't lie down on the bed though – I've made that mistake before too soon after eating and it causes bad indigestion. I decide to organise all my recipes into a folder but I find I can't concentrate enough. I know I need to rest because I nearly trip over as I walk towards the cupboard to get them even though as a precaution, we have put away all the floor rugs to make it safer. I've learnt that while the treatments are going on it's incredibly easy to cause yourself an injury, whether it be tripping over your own feet as you walk around your house on perfectly flat floors or swallowing a tablet too quickly and then it gets stuck and won't go up or down because the water gets trapped in your throat causing you a few moments of real panic, or else picking something up without thinking such as a plate or cup and hurting your finger on the side of it – all sorts of things you never usually think about. You have to try to be alert all the time and be right in the present moment, aware of everything you're doing which is another irony because my brain has never felt so woolly. I probably shouldn't be pushing myself to do things anyway: "Stop being so hard on yourself," my sister said to me earlier. I decide to sit in a comfortable chair and close my eyes. That's enough for now.

8.00pm

I feel distorted. My eyes feel like they're in the wrong part of my face and my cheeks feel swollen. When I look at myself in the mirror, I look all wrong too but my eyesight has been compromised so I'm not sure about what I'm seeing. I ask John if I look distorted. He says, "No, you look like yourself but more tired." I know John doesn't want to upset me, the sweet man that he is, so I can't fully rely on what he's saying. "Do I look puffy?" I ask. "Yes," he replies. "Puffier than usual?" I persist. "You probably feel like that but you look like you – just tired and struggling," and by John putting it in the nicest possible way, I know how bad I really look.

John has bought me some different cordials to try as I'm finding it hard to drink anything including water because everything tastes too horrible. He has bought one that happens to look exactly the same red colour as the Epirubicin Chemo drug. I don't want to tell John that I can't bear to look at it. I put it in the back of the pantry at the very bottom where I can't see it and try for hours to forget about it but I can't. I finally have to tell John to please get rid of it as it reminds me too much of the intravenous drug that causes me so much suffering. Later, a couple on T.V. are drinking a red, alcoholic drink in fancy glasses and I have to look away. Now someone else in a film is drinking wine out of a red-coloured glass. This is a hideous side-effect I hadn't envisaged. I hope I can eventually get past this as it is ruining my peace of mind in a way I wasn't expecting.

4/2/2019 Monday 4.10am

If I had to describe how I feel through all this in one word to sum it up, I would say, "determined" because I have a goal which is to get through the treatment – and now I can actually see the end of it on the calendar as I tick off the days. After that, it's up to me to recover and make the most of my life. How do I want it to be the same? How do I want it to be different? Obviously, it's got to be different, for following the same path and the same thought patterns logically leads to this again and I don't want any more of this.

I know it's not as simple as that but some changes need to be made and for me, they are subtle, internal changes of letting go of the past and letting go of overdoing it in caring about other people and worrying about their problems. I think this is where I have been expending a lot of energy that doesn't actually help anyone and ultimately causes illness to me. It's like a nurturing that's going nowhere and becomes a self-destructive thing eating away at me. I want to be more peaceful and centred on my own life and stop worrying about things I can't do anything about and which people don't want to change anyway, no matter what they say.

In the meantime, I had a horrible day yesterday with terrible indigestion, diarrhoea, lack of energy and almost no voice. It could have been due to a seemingly insignificant thing that I ate – a small potato cake. My sister made a little batch and they looked delicious as they always are but not for me this time – there was a tiny pinch of saffron in the batter but it's a spice and spice does not go with Chemo no matter how minuscule an amount as I found out with pepper a month and a half ago. Bland – all food must be bland or you pay for it with hours of discomfort and pain. It's no good masking all pain and reactions with strong pain killers because then you never find out what's causing it. Give yourself enough time to find out first even if you have to put up with some discomfort because it's the only real way you can prevent it from happening again.

I've always tried to get to the bottom of any trouble in my body as it's always been very sensitive to all chemicals, including perfumes and face creams which quickly result in headaches for me. I have learnt to steer away from all sorts of so-called medications which often leave me feeling far worse off than the original problem. Because I've never had to take much medication for anything, I am very aware of any side-effects particular medicines have on me, including some cholesterol management tablets that caused me depression and anxiety. It took me a long time to work this out as it does with anything that doesn't manifest in a physical way but it was spot on because a different brand didn't have the same effect at all, although it caused bad indigestion instead.

Another thing I've discovered at the moment which leads to physical distress and which is preventable: don't sit for too long, especially on the couch or sofa where you're hunched over a bit as it causes very painful cramping just under the breasts and the upper stomach area. If it happens, get up and stretch your arms up to the ceiling and stretch your torso a few times. Do it in stages and wait for the pain to pass and you might be lucky enough to do a few burps, tiny though they might be, which will let out the pent-up air caused by squashing down on your middle for too long.

I want to be an observer of my body and notice the reaction it has to everything I take – food, drink and medication, that way I can feel as well as possible in this body that needs to last me a lifetime – this extremely sensitive body which is just the way it's always been. I can't do anything about that but I can help it as much as possible. That's why this process I have to go through is so ironic – I never even take an aspirin for headaches and have been lucky enough not to need to mostly and now suddenly I have to undergo the harshest of treatments. It's as though I've said, "Yes, back up the truck full of chemicals and give them all to me intravenously over many months. That's what I want!" It's insane!

5/2/2019 Tuesday

I feel very sick and weak today. Have about a third of my hair left now. The scalp is exposed with a bit of fuzz over it with still some hair at the sides and front. I don't feel good in the stomach or anywhere. I hope this sick feeling lifts away. I feel absolutely revolting.

6/2/2019 Wednesday 5.45am

Feel yucky in the stomach waking up but otherwise okay. Slept till 3.00am and rested and dozed the rest of the night so had a restful, good night. I try to say a positive affirmation: "I allow myself to feel good as I step out of bed and into a new, happy day."

2.00pm

The last days have been very hard – a lot of fatigue, dazed, horrible stomach and mouth.

7/2/2019 Thursday

When food and drink which are part of life's greatest joys can no longer be pleasurable, it's very hard to get through a day. You know you have to eat and drink to keep going – to stay alive but everything tastes repulsive and even before you put anything into your mouth, there's a terrible taste there that won't go away and your stomach feels revolting all the time. But it's temporary – remind yourself it's temporary. Soon all this will be over and you can make a new life for yourself. Of course, the pressure is to slot back into your old life and into the old patterns and ways of thinking and do what you've always done before – and some people may want to do that and good on them, but I want to do something different. If I do exactly the same thing with exactly the same thoughts, won't I end up in exactly the same place? Logic tells me I will. I've had enough of this. I want to be free of many things after this – free in my mind and not waste energy on useless worries and anxieties about the past or the future or get entangled in endless problems that are often not really problems at all if I would just make the decision to go forward. But it's hard to go forward. Most of us so easily get stuck in the past and in the quagmire of regrets and resentment and guilt.

LIFE LESSON:
TAKE AN HONEST LOOK AT YOUR LIFE

Reflect on the things in your life you would like to do differently and begin to take small steps in the direction you'd like to go.

8/2/2019 Friday

Yesterday morning I was at one of my very lowest points – energy was 0-2 on a scale of 10 and I could hardly walk or move at all. I didn't know where to go from there and was thinking to phone the specialist but I knew she would probably say, "Come in to emergency." I thought I'd wait an hour or so to see if I felt any better before I did that. My sister dropped in and saw I was at a very low ebb. She had "The Secret", a book I had already read and given to her ages ago. She told me it fell off the shelf and opened at a page she wanted me to look at. I didn't care much and said I'd do it later. She also suggested I take an anti-nausea tablet which I hadn't thought of doing. I took it straight away. When you're feeling low, you're also not thinking straight. After Maria left, the tablet started to take effect and I felt just slightly better. I looked at the book and the page marked – p.128 "Cathy Goodman 'A Personal Story'." She had been diagnosed with breast cancer. I read the paragraph and then read a couple more pages and realised I was originally thinking like that in a positive way but now had spiralled down into feeling really sick and depressed. I began doing affirmations which I thought were totally false because I didn't feel: "I am healthy", "I am well" – I felt the opposite. But I kept saying things such as: "My body is healing", "Every moment I feel better" – all afternoon on and off until I honestly felt a shift.

By the evening I was feeling more like myself and not just a toxic blob of chemicals which I've been feeling. I could watch TV and enjoy some of it. I laughed during the program, "Would I Lie to You?" and John said, "It's good to hear you laughing." I still felt yucky and I still feel yucky now. How else can you feel during Chemo? But I'm okay again. I can forge ahead. I can see the end in sight and I know I'm on the home stretch now. I just have to remain strong and courageous and not get pulled under by the physical distress. I need to keep strong in my mind – to have mental fortitude – and know that this will soon be over. It's only temporary and I will be better than ever with a healthier mindset and a healthier body.

9/2/2019 Saturday

Had a restful night – dozing a bit but had a stomach ache – I think this is to do with wind. I have to be even more careful about every single thing I eat. I'm eating very little but then I'm not moving a lot either. I have a walk with John each day – just behind our place there's a nice path to a park, about a fifteen minute walk. I also walk up and down our big yard two or three or more times if I can. I do my breast after-surgery exercises. I do other movements inside while listening to a music CD and try to join in with some of the singing. All these things I do daily to help myself as much as I can even though I'd rather not move an inch and can barely drag myself through it sometimes.

My temperature yesterday afternoon was 38.4. I've been told I need to go into emergency if it's over 38 degrees but I waited and did a few things like taking a cool shower, having a Panadol, resting and waiting an hour. It eventually came down to 37.6 so that saved us a lot of work, worry and hassle.

Today I will keep a better eye on it and also make sure that my food is nothing but the plainest which I've been doing all along, but sometimes I'll have an extra mouthful and my stomach can't cope with it. I've got to look after myself the way I look after other people; if I can do that, I'll be a lot better off. In the last days I've realised just how good I am at looking after others. It seems to come naturally to me. I can intuit their wants and needs and make sure they're comfortable and well looked after, though I've come to understand in recent years that this is unusual. I've also realised that my sister and brothers are the same as I am in this way – maybe it's because our mum was often sick throughout our lives. John, who is a wonderful human being is finding it hard most of the time to know what I want and I have found I'm no good at telling him or anyone else – I don't want to put them out. So really the problem is with me: I've never had to be the sick one. This is an incredibly different and difficult role for me and I'm hating it. I try to be gracious and understanding, but a few times now I've quietly lost my temper and been annoyed that the thing I asked for wasn't bought or found or available. I know I'm not being fair at all and it's not like me but sometimes I feel so fed up. Again, I know I have to change that - instead of being angry, annoyed and resentful, I need to communicate clearly what I want and not expect others to read my mind or figure it out.

11/2/2019 Monday

I feel like I'm crawling on all fours just to get to the finish line – which for me is the last Chemo treatment.

12/2/2019 Tuesday 4.05pm

I have been battling with a chest infection again and on antibiotics three times a day but they're giving me a rash. I've contacted the specialist who has advised me to continue on them unless the rash gets worse. This cough needs to lift. I don't know where I am anymore. I just feel hemmed in by everything – everywhere hurts and I almost can't cope. But I know I'm near the finish line with all this. Be brave! Be strong! Courage! Courage! Courage! Just one more treatment. You can do it!

I just feel at such a low ebb but I'm going outside now to walk in the backyard and do some movement to help my body get better. I can crumple in a heap later if needs be or maybe this chest thing will miraculously be cured.

13/2/2019 Wednesday 6.00pm

I have to go in to emergency as my temperature is going haywire at 39.8.

The two nurses try not to show that my temperature is a concern as it is far too high. I feel a bit dazed. It looks like I won't be going back home tonight.

For the first three days in hospital my temperature remains very high and I have night sweats so that the sheets and pillow slips and my hospital gown all have to be changed in the middle of the night as they are soaking wet. It is uncomfortable and annoying and sometimes happens two and three times a night – not the full bed strip for the nurses have put down something else which is hotter and more unpleasant for me but it prevents the perspiration soaking through the sheets. My night gowns still have to be changed though.

The nurses are good, but for me those minutes of sitting in the wet hospital gown feel like hours and I am cold and shivering by the time a nice clean, warm one is placed over my shoulders. I feel embarrassed about it all and one night when one nurse is on her own, I help her make the bed as I feel I have been a lot of trouble.

I have to be given so many blood tests that eventually not enough blood comes out to fill the tube. Every vein that can be accessed has been punctured – all from my left arm as my right arm can't be used because of the breast surgery and the removal of the lymph node. The tops of my feet are used which is more painful but still not enough blood can be removed. My arm with the constant drip needle is also becoming extremely sore and looking like it's on the verge of becoming a problem so I just can't wait for the moment I no longer need any more of the antibiotics my body has been pumped with since the first day I was admitted.

20/2/2019 Wednesday

I have finally come home after being in hospital for six days and six nights –diagnosed with A-typical Pneumonia, which means an unusual type of Pneumonia.

21/2/2019 Thursday

Being at home is so good it's like a dream that I feel I might wake up from. The six days in hospital felt like six weeks or at times even six months but I came out of there feeling more grateful than ever. There are so many people with such worse illnesses and situations who can't go back to their homes or can't walk as the cancer becomes progressively worse. I was in an oncology ward for the last couple of days and was very lucky to be in with some lovely ladies: Leah, who had a very loving family and who was full of love herself and Christina who had no family except a nephew and had been in hospital for over a month and Effie who lived alone and had been through breast cancer which she considered not too bad compared to the cancer she contracted after that and the other treatments involved. Silvia was 92 and had suffered a fall. She knew she wasn't going home and although she was resigned about it, she said to me wistfully: "I'd love to go home but I know I won't be going back to my house." She would be returning to a nursing home although she was very alert and articulate.

22/2/2019 Friday

Having had pneumonia has left me weak. I have quite a few bruises on my arm and feet from where the needles have been and any movement of my left arm is painful. The top of my left hand looks different too: one of the veins is raised more than it was before and another one looks like a miniature sausage – all bumpy with troughs and valleys.

26/2/2019 Tuesday

The day after final Chemo session – don't feel good in the stomach or the mouth. Very off food and drink. Can't wait to get through all of this and feel better.

27/2/2019 Wednesday

So everything still goes on – forcing myself to eat and drink – the right things too so I can feel better quicker – Weeties, porridge and prune juice. I took my two Coloxyl and Senna tablets last night to get things moving so that terrible constipation doesn't happen again that requires the emergency department and an enema. Apart from that I feel okay. The Chemo is still in my system but the treatments are over and every time I go to the toilet I get rid of some of the toxins.

I know it's time to be stronger than ever now to get over these last hurdles and though I feel weary I've got to muster up the strength and not give up.

28/2/2019 Thursday

Last day of summer with 37 degree heat. It was tough today. I felt weak and sick in the stomach with a horrible taste in my mouth but I know that's all part of it because I've taken all my tablets including the anti-nausea one. It's only three days since the Chemo treatment although it feels like three weeks so I mustn't be impatient – all is going well. I've been resting and doing my meditation and exercises and also little jobs around the house here and there. John has been working hard – there's been no rain for ages so the garden needs water and there's lots to do inside too. I try to help where I can but I know at the moment the best way I can help is to get better as soon as possible – I'm getting there. I am eating and drinking carefully though I don't want any and doing all my tedious mouth washes four times a day and everything I've been advised to do to make things better for me. The saliva in my mouth has mostly dried up – this happened from the beginning of the treatments and has become progressively worse - and it means all food is sticking fiendishly to my teeth so the mouth washes are necessary. This is another of the nasty side-effects of the treatments and as per the instruction booklet, I've had no crunchy foods whatsoever from the beginning because I certainly don't want my teeth falling out. John phoned our dentist of over thirty years, Doctor Peter Wellington, for advice about my teeth after the first Chemo session, when the ulcers started to be a problem. I count him as part of the wonderful team of medical experts who look after us which includes our general practitioner, John's heart specialist, and my three oncology specialists. I trust and admire these people. Peter's advice, which I have paid strict attention to, was to take extra care with flossing, brushing manually and keeping up the mouth washes as these things are extra important during Chemo to maintain dental health.

I'm getting all the help I can get and I receive it all gratefully. I know how lucky I am to have all this support from really great people. It's still hard to get through each day but I know I'm one of the luckiest and I will make the most of this opportunity. I'm going to take this second go at life with both hands and enjoy it more than ever before.

1/3/2019 Friday

Have felt rotten this morning. Started well, then the tide turned and I went into a slump. Hands and feet hot, hard to drink water without choking, a strong pain high in the chest like a blockage then the onset of a migraine, have a horrible, sickly taste in my mouth and at the back of my throat all the time and feel dizzy too. Nearly fainted at the table this afternoon I was so dizzy – my head was spinning. Maybe it was the heat. Had a bit of a panic for a moment; it was such a horrible feeling – as though everything was going totally out of control – luckily John was sitting right next to me so I held onto his arm and closed my eyes and it finally passed. Had a partial migraine again after my eye received a stab of light reflecting off something outside. Ready to take anti-reflux medication.

After two hours of resting on the bed I've started to feel better. It's another hot, 37 degree day so the heat doesn't help, but overall I'm okay right now. It's good to know the bad times pass - those awful symptoms lift away – not all of them but slowly they will. I've been doing Havening, Tapping and Meditation – all help a bit but the chemicals are all too harsh to make the discomfort and pain lift away completely. Any alleviation is better than nothing though.

Everyone says I'm brave but I don't feel brave. I just feel that I have to put one foot in front of the other and keep going. The alternative is to give up and that's no good. It's been a very tough day – not feeling well at all. Looking forward to a much better day tomorrow. Just keep going – every day must get better. My body wants to heal and I will help it as much as I can. I'm in good hands with all the doctors who are helping me. I believe a tiny dose of hope is better than the best of medicine taken with despair. I'm forever hopeful – it's in my nature – after all my Maiden name was Speranza which means Hope so I can't help being hopeful – I can't be anything else – that's what I am - that's who I am.

Recently I've seen a program called *Miriam's Deathly Adventure* which I've loved watching. In it the marvellous Miriam Margolyes explores death and dying in her humorous, down-to-earth and very real way. When a teenage cancer patient says, "Isn't it hope that kills us?" Miriam's inspirational response is, "It is not hope that kills us …. hope keeps you going. Hope is the chink in the curtain that lets the light through," and I want to add another part of Leonard Cohen's *Anthem* here: "There is a crack in everything – that's how the light gets in." I agree that the weakest part of us can become the strongest part of us. It's our vulnerability that gives us a direct link to the divine.

2/3/2019 Saturday

Having another very weak day today – can hardly walk around without feeling like I might topple over. Maybe a rest will fix it. I'll try.

Feel terrible today – furry in the mouth and throat with horrible taste – very weak and just generally revolting. I want it to pass and be over and done with – I've had enough now. I feel really sick.

It's time for me to feel better now and I'm ready to be healthy and well.

3/3/2019 Sunday

Stomach ache this morning and been to the toilet twice. Mouth is furry and so is throat. I don't want to take tablets – they make things worse in so many ways. If only I can get through this patch and feel well. It's time for improvement now – I'm sick of this on every level. I release it all. Take it away from me please Universe. I've had enough. I release it all – this illness, this condition, this disease, this discomfort, this pain, this yuckiness, this horror – whatever it's called, I lift my arms up now and release it all. Please take it away from me forever and for good, everything that doesn't work in my body, everything that's a threat to me, everything that can cause ill health, lift it away from me now please.

4/3/2019 Monday

Everything nearly got the better of me yesterday. I was so weak and feeling so sick and the furry tongue and throat were terrible. Reverted slightly to tears a couple of times but refused to let the frustration and feeling sorry for myself take control so put a stop to it after a little bit. I'm better this morning. Didn't get much sleep but rested and prayed and asked for healing which I got. My eyes are very sensitive to the light now but I am okay. I'm trying to do things differently this morning: had porridge and I'm waiting for the boiled water to cool down rather than drink tap water – hoping it will make a big difference to my mouth and throat. Can it help anyone to know this? I don't know – even if it helps a couple of people, I suppose that's pretty good.

11.25am

What a hard road this is! I have had to page the specialist who has ordered me a mouth medication – drops to swivel and swallow for this fungal problem that won't lift away on its own – but I'm onto it now and on the road to recovery.

5/3/2019 Tuesday

This mouth fungus is proving to be a revolting thing and difficult to shake – but I am dealing with it and I expect a full recovery in the morning because of all the hard work I've done with medication four times a day and meditation and doing everything possible to clear it up.

6/3/2019 Wednesday

It's 29 years since John had the triple bypass operation after the heart attack. What a horrible time that was but John showed me the true meaning of bravery and he rallied and fought and it never stopped him doing anything he needed to do, nor did he ever use it as an excuse not to do things. Then in 2007 he had to have a quadruple bypass. That's what I call brave!

Now in this month, on this afternoon what do I have to say that could be of any use to anyone? I'm feeling very down. This mouth and throat fungus is wearying me and making me feel ghastly. It's all so putrid from beginning to end – I mean the whole thing from the October diagnosis – all revolting and repulsive and makes me want to vomit – in fact it's all I can do to stop myself most of the time. I will tell you what I tell me: "Get through it – get to the other side of it and say, 'I'm having a new life! There was something about that other life that didn't work! I'm going to make new choices. I deserve a happy life. I want a happy life." That makes me wonder, "What do I want to happen? And "What am I going to do to help that to happen? So "What's the first step I need to take to move forward?" Then I have to ask myself, "What would make me happy right now?" That's a hard one. Nothing is appealing at the moment. Maybe a phone call from a friend? It's a tentative question but it has a brave answer – "Well let me call them!"

It's time to take action in my own life. If I want something to be a certain way, I must work towards making that happen. If I don't like the way something is, I must work towards changing it. Enough of this endless thinking and delving and trying to work things out. Maria constantly says to me, "Sis, stop over-analysing everything!" and being the very wise person she is, I know she's right. Over-thinking things often causes me a lot of tension and worry. Time to do! Take one step at a time and watch how things change. "Change" – I have been scared of that word but that was in the past – no more! Now I embrace change for it means life, it means open doors and freedom and happiness. It means choices and me choosing the way I want things to be. It means personal power and me taking charge of my own life. It is mine after all and it's the only one I've got. Everyone has their own and they're not entitled to more than one each - surely that's enough for anyone. Let each person direct his or her own life – that's enough to be getting on with in one lifetime.

Outside it's hailing right now after weeks of no rain. It hardly ever hails – what beautiful music it makes! And now rain follows. It's wonderful! Cleaning, refreshing, cleansing away old, mouldy ideas and thoughts, eradicating stale thinking patterns and ruts I've fallen into over the years. "Let go!" it's saying, "Let go of everything you don't need. Notice all the areas in your body that are holding tension and release it. Notice all the old, stagnant ideas and feelings you keep reverting back to – all the old irritations, fears, resentments and guilt. Let it go. Let it all go for your life's sake! This is an opportunity for a second chance at life. Take it and run with it!"

LIFE LESSON: MAKE A FRESH START

Begin to make changes in the way you think. Don't go back to exactly the way you were doing things before and the way you were thinking about things before. Accept that you are not going to be the same as you were before the cancer and treatment. Don't be afraid of that. Welcome it. If you can be open to change, many things are going to be better - maybe everything. Consciously let go of past hurts, grief, guilt, anger and any other negative feelings. Do this through meditation, prayer, music, exercise and any way that works for you.

Vincent phoned just then as I was writing this and must have tapped into my worries because he said this is a golden opportunity for me – this second chance at life – he is a very spiritual person. He actually said, "Golden opportunity" – could a great message be any clearer?

7/3/2019 Thursday

My mind is trying so hard to stay positive but my body is in a lot of trouble. I don't think anyone could have thought up a worse torture than this last complication of mouth and throat fungus. In my mouth and mostly on my tongue and at the back of my throat and continuing down, I can feel a terrible furriness. This coupled with the Chemo has made it for me the longest week of my life. All the other weeks have been horrendous too but looking at the calendar this time, I just can't believe it's been a week since the last treatment – every day has felt longer than a week – this mouth infection has been so revolting and the medicine I have to take for it four times a day. Repulsive! It makes all food and drink taste even more terrible. Anything that takes away the joy of food and drink, takes away a good part of the joy of living. And that's how it's been for months now and has lately been getting worse instead of better because of all these extra complications.

I just have to try not to give up; it would be easy to do – I feel so weary and worn down. I feel wretched and that's how I've felt throughout this – very, very sick. My body feels wrecked and weak, totally ravaged and destroyed. I am a trembling, puffy, swollen, fuzzy-headed blob of a mess. Every particle of me has been affected, from my toe nails to my eyesight and in a bad, destructive way where I'm trying to hold on, hoping it doesn't go too far so that it can't come back to balance or healing. I'm scared of not being able to find my balance again, of my body not being able to get back to good health again. But I try to trust in the goodness of the Universe. Surely, I won't be deserted now in my greatest hour of need? I don't know. I'm shaken to the core with this illness.

I've seen so clearly throughout this time how many people focus on all the wrong things – on destructive, mean things, instead of on healing and helping each other and eradicating all the diseases and illnesses in the world. We can go into outer space yet Chemo is the best we have against cancer which kills bad and good cells and can kill off the person as well – it's nearly done that to me, particularly in that first week of allergies and horrendous side-effects and reactions. And since then, with no exaggeration, it's been killing my body off by slow degrees. I look twenty years older at least and I'm frail, my hair is wispy and almost non-existent, my eyesight is bad, many days I've hardly got a voice at all and can only talk in a tiny whisper and everything in my mouth is either sickly sweet or bitter even when there's nothing in it. I feel pushed to my limit of resistance and resilience and this had better improve soon or my last bit of strength will be gone - and then I'll be gone.

8/3/2019 Friday 4.40pm

This mouth and throat fungus is proving difficult to shift but John has bought a new medication from the chemist so I will keep persevering as I do about everything and hopefully by the morning this will be gone and I will feel much better as the medicine upsets my stomach as well as everything else. It's time for things to start going more smoothly now and for all the bumps and hiccoughs and hurdles to be behind me. I look forward to a new and brighter day full of good health, peace and happiness.

I've been feeling very, very sick this afternoon – have had bad diarrhoea and just keep feeling worse. John has suggested I ring the oncologist but I've decided to wait till tomorrow. "There's still Friday before the weekend," I said to John. "Today's Friday," said John. "What? Today?" I'm not in my right head at all. I'm shocked that all day I've been thinking it's Thursday. Luckily Emma has sent a prescription to the chemist for a different medication. I have started it and already seen a slight improvement.

9/3/2019 Saturday

Often through other people we discover where we're at or how bad things were in the past during a certain incident and that's what happened to me. Yesterday when I was speaking to Maria, she told me how serious it was for me in that first few weeks of Chemo when my head was completely fuzzy and I didn't really know where I was. "It could have gone either way," Maria said and I really did feel that at the time. I knew I should have been in hospital when all those side-effects and reactions and allergies were raging in my body but I didn't want to go. That first dose which I was very allergic to nearly killed me.

10/3/2019 Sunday

It has been only two weeks since the last treatment and it has honestly felt like two months. I have to keep looking at the calendar to believe it's been such a short time. I look like I've put on weight because I look puffy but I've actually lost five kilos. My hair is three quarters gone.

12/3/2019 Tuesday

I so much want to be well now – I've had enough of sickness. I've been very lucky – I've had lots of people cheering me on. I continue to affirm: "I am well. All is well. I feel fit and healthy. I accept and love myself."

I am beginning to feel more like my old self this afternoon. I am getting better. I can think more clearly. Maybe everything's going to be all right: I will get over this and one day it will be behind me and I will think back at how I was able to get through this terrible thing that devastated my body and nearly killed it off completely and wonder at how I was strong enough to withstand such doses of poison in my system. This has been one of the toughest experiences of my life.

13/3/2019 Wednesday

Don't waste any effort on things that don't matter. Don't be weak in the face of other people's bullying which presents itself in many different and sometimes subtle ways. John and I went to the shops for the shortest time and I wanted to go to see if I could manage it so John went to the post office while I stayed in the supermarket wearing a hat to cover up the baldness and disposable gloves to avoid germs. I made myself as inconspicuous as possible, always on the alert in case anyone was coughing or had a cold so I could keep well away. I was feeling quite dazed and out of kilter under the bright lights but luckily there was hardly anyone around as it was so early.

At the fruit and vegetable section I looked at the bunches of celery not sure whether I wanted one. Another woman was there complaining that they were too big. She wanted me to agree with her so I gave a half nod so as not to have to answer. She called over one of the workers and ordered a half bunch. The man wasn't keen and told her they were being sold as a full bunch today. "They're too big - that lady wants the other half," she said loudly, pointing at me. No, I didn't! I hadn't said any such thing! – but I didn't say that – I was surprised but it was easier to keep quiet. I was merely looking at the bunches of celery when the sly woman quickly saw her chance to get what she wanted by involving me. She had asked for something annoying - half a bunch of celery - so the man had to go into the back and cut it for her, wrap it and find out the price. She was a nuisance and a bully and because I was right there and weak, I got used. But how stupid and weak was I? "No, I don't want half," I should have spoken up and said, "You wear it! You're asking for something difficult – you take the responsibility for it instead of putting it onto somebody else just to justify your own selfish demands to that poor worker." I would never have been so rude as that but I didn't need to be. I simply needed to stand up for myself. Again, I find it easier to stand up for others if I see an injustice but when it comes to myself, I'm still allowing others to take advantage of me. It was another example of my weakness in not speaking up and I was disappointed in myself. I did go back and get a full bunch of celery anyway and put back the half that I hadn't requested. I knew someone else would be grateful for it but it didn't stop me feeling angry with myself for not speaking up earlier and for continuing a pattern which I had been given an opportunity to break. It's pretty clear that all the resolutions in the world aren't going to change anything unless I'm willing to take that first step to move forward and really look after myself.

14/3/2019 Thursday

Getting better all the time now. Trying some new foods and going okay – still having diarrhoea but I think it's because of the anti-fungal medication – that's still going but it's nearly over – I hope!

18/3/2019 Monday 5.35am

After four days of starting to feel better, this morning has been horrible. I've been going over the same old rubbish that I used to do and had over an hour of sleeplessness so I decided to get up. I'm seeing the surgeon today for a check-up. I thought I was past going down the same old negative tracks, but obviously not. It can happen very easily again. I don't like it and I don't like the pressures that come with day-to-day living.

I need a new way of thinking if I'm not going to repeat old patterns, but how do I think differently and be true to myself? I know it's no good going over old stuff but it still seems to happen.

19/3/2019 Tuesday

I learned one thing today by watching cancer sufferer, Professor Randy Pausch's lecture online and then his wife being interviewed. Her mantra: "Not helpful" is a good one to use when going down negative tracks or when negative thoughts creep in which are not helpful in any way. To see such a positive, intelligent man so full of life and youth talking candidly about dying is a sobering and uplifting experience. It reminds me to be grateful for every moment of my life and not to allow negativity and lack of love or lack of forgiveness to weigh me down even for one moment. Life is good and I can make it even better – it's in my power to make my day happy, fun and full of joy and laughter. It's up to me to choose the things I want to do and see the people I want to see and spend time with. After all, my time is finite so it's very precious. I'd love to be more light-hearted so I might need to work on that by choosing better and not allowing negativity to use up my time and energy.

20/3/2019 Wednesday

It's the small things that matter – that's what has been confirmed to me today. I have felt like whistling – whistling! And I've actually been whistling on and off. I never thought I'd feel like whistling or singing again. After loving to sing all my life it's been hard not having a voice even to speak with most of the time throughout these months – and a completely tuneless voice when it has reappeared.

I have enjoyed my lunch at Maria's – I could smell the delicious food as John and I walked up to her door. And there was a huge patch of time when I couldn't smell anything at all and detested the taste of everything – even water. During the past three days I have had some chocolate, cheese, nuts, a crunchy raw chestnut – very carefully - and I've been able to drink water properly without choking. These are all things I haven't been able to do for months. I can hardly believe it's all coming back.

I can't think properly yet and I'm not making the connection with some very obvious things such as putting certain foods on my plate unless I see someone else doing it first. For example, I saw Maria putting the homemade giardiniera onto her plate rather than straight onto the bread as I had been trying to do, spilling oil on the tablecloth, but it hadn't even occurred to me that it was possible to put it onto my plate first. When Maria did it I thought it was such an inspired idea. "Yeah, that's a much better way of doing it," I said feeling as though she'd invented something completely new and fabulous that I could never come up with myself.

I really hope my brain can be all right again after the Chemo. I know my body is in ruins so why should my brain remain unharmed? - after all, the Chemo affects every white cell of your body. Both John and Maria as well as Vincent and Lorrie often say to me that I'm doing a great job which I don't believe I am at all. John says, "You've been through a life-threatening thing," and Maria says, "There were times when I didn't think you'd make it; you were in a really bad way, so don't worry about that – you're alive – that's all that matters." This helps me so much but I mustn't let it go to my head – it's giving me leeway to be a selfish, lazy and self-absorbed idiot. I have to remind myself that I want to come out of this a better, more balanced person rather than a cantankerous, self-centred tyrant who uses illness as the excuse for being impossible. I might allow it for a little while though!

I am absolutely astounded at what a wonderful creation the body is. At every moment it is ready to heal, to be well, to be the healthiest it can be and with the slightest effort from us it goes forward in leaps and bounds. It lets us know what it needs to be at its optimum; it tells us through pain and discomfort what's wrong and what it doesn't need – if we will only listen. It wants to be well, to function at its highest capacity. Our body is the vessel that houses us –the very essence of us – and it does this in the perfect way if we will let it. Even when we throw poisons into it, whether they are drugs or alcohol or poor choices of food and drink, it tries to work through this and find a way to keep functioning – it might be by vomiting or diarrhoea just to re-establish some sort of balance again. For the first time in my life, I have gained complete respect for this amazing vessel that carries me around: I am in awe of my body for what it has put up with over these last months and how it is recovering after being so wrecked and tormented.

**LIFE LESSON:
CHOOSE TO STAY POSITIVE**

Don't fret about getting better or worry about whether it will ever happen – it's a waste of energy. Our bodies are amazing: while there's breath in us, our bodies will keep healing. The way you can help is to stay as positive as you can and believe things will improve. Be aware of negative thoughts and don't give them free reign; instead, replace them with positive affirmations.

21/3/2019 Thursday

I heard this morning on the radio that a tablet has been developed which can dissolve leukemia - wonderful!

I know that the time must come when there will be an easier, better, quicker way of helping to eradicate cancer than Chemotherapy that destroys the cancer cells but also destroys the good cells and therefore the body. For the body to then take months if not years to recover from a treatment that offers a tiny percentage of hope that the cancer won't return is terrible, but when you're facing death, you will undergo any treatment that is available even with the slimmest chance of success.

I know there are and have been countless people who have endured much longer Chemotherapy treatment than I have and so much worse in the past, some with almost no chance of success and I'm not saying all this to whinge and complain when I've had it easy compared to many, but I say it to state as a fact and to add that as human beings we need to improve things in this area. Although we've come a long way, it needs to be much better and people shouldn't have to be put through these horrendous therapies to give them an extra 15% chance of the cancer not reappearing. It's a terrible thing to put a person through and at the moment it's the best thing we've got. This is the best we've got? I ask myself in disbelief – in 2019? – When we can go to the moon and land a robot on Mars.

When I saw Julia, my surgeon for a final check-up, I asked her if she had any advice for me about the cancer not coming back. She wasn't expecting the question and said she didn't really have any advice except: don't smoke, drink only a little and stay positive. I don't drink or smoke so those two are easy and I think that mostly I've been a positive person all my life – but *staying* positive is a different matter – that's not so easy especially in the last years with the sudden death of my brother and the difficulty of finalising his will. My sister and I were the executors and there were a lot of complications to deal with even though he didn't actually own all that much and he had mortgages but we had to do the best we could for his two much loved daughters. When I told them about the cancer and the treatments I would have to begin as soon as possible - after the initial expressions of shock and alarm, Bridgette said resolutely, "Just tell me whatever you need me to do around the house and I can come and help," and Gail said to me confidently, "Dad will be with you every step of the way," so I could relax - between them, Anthony's two sweethearts had it all covered.

Anyway, the staying positive can be a hurdle as I have found myself crying a lot over the past three and a half years. A couple of years ago, on one of our visits to John's heart specialist, Doctor Tremain said something I've never forgotten because of the clever pun and because it was so true. When I told him we try to live a peaceful life and avoid stress as much as possible but that we were finding it hard to stay clear of it altogether he said, "You can't by-pass life." In other words, you can't completely avoid stress. That made me realise that of course you can't because it's part of life but you have to learn to manage it and not let it take over.

Counting today, it is 95 days since I started Chemo – just over three months and today I had a toasted ciabatta roll with cheese and tomato for the first time since I began the treatment. It wasn't as delicious as I remembered it but then my tastebuds aren't the same as they were. I still enjoyed the process of having it even though three hours later it ended up giving me diarrhoea – probably because of the cheese, which reminded me that I'm not back to normal yet. I was pretty good though to be able to have it in the first place and to be out for over an hour.

22/3/2019 Friday

John has told me today and a few other times too that he is so proud of me for being so brave in getting through everything. He said: "I don't think I could have done it." He is wonderful but I've told him I don't feel brave at all – I've just been doing what had to be done; trudging on, moving forward, hoping I could continue to endure. "A lot of people give up," John said. "I don't blame them," I answered, "it's really hard to keep going – when you have gone into it feeling well and you get sicker and sicker – in that first three weeks I wondered what I was doing and whether I was doing the right thing. There were times during the three months when I truly thought I may not make it. My sister and brother and everyone I knew said they felt it was the right thing for me sometimes in a very intense tone that made me listen and remember. And I knew before all that it was the right path for me so I had to continue on. I could hear my brothers, Anthony and Vincent in my head saying, "Get on with it!" in the funny way they'd call out if someone was faffing around or making a convoluted speech.

It was the full support of family and friends that kept me going even when I faltered or was too sick to know what to do. It was a friend of mine, Kim, who originally mentioned the waterfall meditation she had heard about in an email when I said that I was feeling so dreadfully hot due to the treatments. I couldn't find any on the internet that really suited me and eventually it was Lorrie who gave me her own waterfall meditation which I did often under the shower because it was as simple as: "Imagine you are under a cleansing waterfall which washes away all the lower energy, emotions and situations that no longer serve you. Say, 'I let go of all this negative energy and I feel refreshed and energised." And she also said, "Just make up your own one." Friends sent me emails with great affirmations, poems and inspirational thoughts. Everyone I knew sent me get well texts and said encouraging things like, "You've got this Grace!" "You can do it!" to strengthen my resolve, while the prayers of all my extended family were pouring in as well as those of all our friends.

I've been very lucky – even though I haven't seen anyone except my sister, I know everyone has kept away because that's what we wanted, but they have kept in touch through phone calls, texts and emails, cards and good wishes through other members of family and friends because they knew I didn't have the energy to keep up with anyone and John was busy looking after me.

Dad has been gone a long time now but I often remember some of his sayings. One old Italian proverb he sometimes used to quote was: "Everyone cries with their own eyes." It can mean: "Others have their own problems that's why they don't care much about ours" or "People are only aware of their own problems and pain and they don't understand yours unless they go through the same thing themselves". In other words, you can only fully know about your own pain. I think if we use our imagination and empathy no one needs to be alone in their suffering. As sentient human beings, we have the power to really help each other overcome dire circumstances. My family and friends have proved this - they have all helped me to make it through the most difficult time in my life and I know I couldn't have done it without them.

23/3/2019 Saturday

This is something I've learned in the last months through my own experience: when you find out someone has cancer if you want to be helpful then don't be dismissive – don't pretend it's nothing; don't tell them stories about people who have had it far worse than you – of course there are millions of those; don't be in floods of tears either – none of that helps. But it does help to have someone who's for you and strong by your side. If you want to be a true friend, start with this intention – just have it as a thought in your head: "I don't pretend to know the pain you feel, but I'm here for you, to help in whatever way I can, in whatever way is helpful to you, even if that means waiting to see you after all the treatments are over."

Part 2

Radiation Treatment

26/3/2019 Tuesday

Yesterday I had to go in to the St John of God Berwick Hospital for a scan in preparation for the Radiation treatments. I hadn't thought about this much at all leading up to the day as it was enough to get through the Chemo. It was always at the back of my mind, but getting measured up, having a 'map' drawn over my chest and speaking to the nurses made it all very real and I felt nervous. This was a big deal and they had to get it exactly right. I was going to be given nineteen sessions starting from the 4th of April. I knew I was in good hands but by the end of it I was feeling a bit scared. As I returned to the area where I needed to change out of my hospital gown, I smiled at a lady waiting her turn and she smiled back. Soon we introduced ourselves. Shirley told me she had had a double mastectomy and had already been given nine treatments. "It's as though I haven't had anything," she said. "Don't listen to all the stories. Everyone's different but I haven't felt anything." I suddenly felt relieved to hear something positive.

She was a very alert little lady between 75 and 85 and completely tuned in to how I was feeling. I was trying to help her feel better but she helped me instead. "You look healthy; you'll be fine," she said. "I was very healthy before I had the Chemo," I said. "Now you're smiling again," she said happily and repeated, "don't listen to all the stories." I didn't know I hadn't been smiling so that was a surprise and I realised I had been looking very serious. We wished each other well with the hope that we might see each other again over the next treatments.

27/3/2019 Wednesday

Went to Cabrini Hospital for my lung scan today. It was all easy and I think everything is fine with my lungs now and I'm fully recovered from the pneumonia so I feel good about that. We picked up the prescription for the mouth fungus and that's a relief so that now I can get rid of it once and for all. We also bought the cream I need to help prevent burns during the Radiation treatments - a new medication called Strata XRT which my specialist has suggested I try. All in all we had a good day and I'm feeling better. Tomorrow Vincent and Lorrie arrive from Queensland and I can't wait to see them.

We are going to have a great get-together for Maria's birthday during their stay so I am able to see all my extended family. I'm glad the party gives them an opportunity to see for themselves I am okay – not my usual self - but with a positive mind-set about making a good recovery.

6/4/2019 Saturday

Vincent and Lorrie have come and gone and we had a wonderful week together catching up and having a few laughs. Just being with them made me feel better. They stayed with my sister who lives close by so I was able to see them every day even though I had to get back home after a couple of hours each visit because of the fatigue that seems to sneak in slyly. My voice also tends to give up as well and I begin coughing after a bit of talking. Despite all that and needing to have the toilet close by, I still loved spending time with them and began missing them as soon as they boarded the shuttle bus which came by to pick them up to take them to the airport. I tried not to be too upset because I knew we'd continue to keep in touch with the telephone but still, it's hard not to see them for months and sometimes years at a time.

It was also a chance to see all of my beautiful and loving nieces and nephews and partners so it was a big occasion. I hadn't seen them for months and I'm sure they could see changes in me but I could also see changes in them. They all seemed so grown up. It was Maria's birthday so a good chance to kick up our heels. Not that I was doing anything as energetic as that but it was great to celebrate my beautiful sister's birthday and have Vincent and Lorrie there as well. I wasn't able to do a lot of talking because of my weak voice - which some of them might have been thankful for - but it was good to catch up with everyone even for an hour or two before John and I left the party and went home.

After we waved off Vincent and Lorrie and brushed away the tears, I had to focus on my treatment program immediately as I was up to the next stage after Chemo. I started Radiation Treatment that same afternoon.

3.30pm

I haven't wanted to think too much about this treatment so I don't dwell on it when it comes into my thoughts. This last week has taken my mind off it anyway as my sister and John and I have tried to spend as much time with Vincent and Lorrie as we can. We saw them off at 1.30pm and two hours later I'm ready for my first treatment – not ready really, but there at the clinic. The nurses ask me how I feel – "A bit nervous," I answer, and they say happily that it's a normal response to something unknown and like this. The truth is I'm really scared but I don't want to worry John. I'm determined to brave it out and not show how worried I am about it all. The nurses and Radiation therapists are magnificent – all young women and a couple of young men, knowledgeable and compassionate. They explain every step of the procedure, calmly and confidently. I have to lie on a hard, narrow bed underneath a monster of a machine that takes time to position, although the procedure itself is only seven minutes long.

10/4/2019 Wednesday

I've had my fifth radiation treatment and all is going okay. I spoke to two other people in the waiting area today. Joan was having her last treatment. She seemed to be about ten years older than me, had daughters and many grandchildren so that kept her strong. Simon might have been in his early fifties and had cancer which affected the male organs but he wasn't specific. He asked us if we got depressed at any time. We both said no and Joan gave the above as her reason. I qualified mine with: "Not exactly – I've never felt I want to jump out of the window, but I have felt sad and scared at times."

We all admitted it was a big shock to learn we had cancer. Simon said he had tears running down his cheeks when the doctor told him he was in stage three.

Joan said, "If anyone in my family was going to have to have it then I'd rather it was me." Surprisingly, I had felt the same and said so. "I've always listened to my body," she said. I said, "I have too and I've always been my own doctor," I added. We agreed that we couldn't do that this time and that we'd got to where we were, having had very healthy lives up till then but now we were in other people's hands and had to rely on them. We were strangers but our thought processes were similar. "This is too serious," I said. "We need help with getting well this time – we have needed surgery and all these other treatments. We have to trust they know what they're doing."

Again, I went away from those conversations feeling very grateful: Simon had to have thirty-nine treatments and Joan, twenty-six. My nineteen were easier to cope with though it had sounded so many before now – and Joan was travelling from the country to come here every day, while for me it was less than twenty minutes away. Simon was alone, separated from his wife, while I have John who supports me and has been helping me throughout all this.

It appears that nothing much is happening during the treatments but today I have felt a lot of heat in my right breast and it is hot to the touch whereas the other side is much cooler.

12/4/2019 Friday

There's a bell along the corridor on the way to the Radiation waiting room. I hadn't noticed it till I was told about it by Joan and Simon yesterday. Simon had asked us if we were going to ring the bell and I asked, "What bell?" Joan said she wasn't going to because it wouldn't be over for five more years, when and if the body is declared free of cancer, but I disagree. I think it's good to have small goals and reach them. I have found that to be a good approach for me as I've inched my way forward and put each difficult thing behind me. And when I finish all the Radiation treatments, that will be an achievement and worthy of celebration – with the ringing of a bell at least. Five years is a long way away and I prefer to believe I will definitely be free of all cancer as soon as the final treatment is over.

My hair looks very raggedy but there are more important things going on right now and my woollen beanies from the Reject Shop are doing a good job when I am out of the house occasionally. I still prefer to stay at home as people have colds and sniffles and I want to keep away from any chance of catching the bad flu that's all over the news – I don't think my body could cope with that at all right now.

13/4/2019 Saturday

I have finally been able to wear my earrings today after many days. I've been dealing with an earlobe infection – something I wasn't expecting and it took three or four days before I realised it was getting steadily worse instead of better after trying everything I knew to clear it up. It's been red, swollen and painful and I couldn't get my earring in at all. I knew the hole would close up if this went on and I couldn't see myself getting my ears pierced again so I went to see the chemist. He told me to use an antiseptic solution on it four times a day which should clear it up. I had been using it once a day as I've always done for any small infections but obviously at the moment that's not effective enough. He was correct in his diagnosis and advice because I did as he suggested and my earlobe infection is well and truly over.

I have to be much, much kinder to myself even though I'm better than I ever was in this regard. I've just realised the cream I need to put on around the breast area needs to be done in a gentler way as the whole area is very tender now and sensitive to the touch after seven treatments. And truthfully, I would put the cream on far more carefully if I was doing it for someone else and that tells me I need to take more care of myself and stop thinking of myself as less important than everyone else.

7.10pm

I feel sad that my brother is in Queensland and I hardly ever see him but I know that's where his life is and has been for nearly thirty years so it's nothing new. But now I feel there's not much time left for all of us and life is very short. I have been speaking to him on the phone every day since all this started so I suppose that's one of the hidden blessings of this serious condition. Another one is that I will try to look out for myself more and try not to get too upset about other people's problems. I can see much more clearly now that many of our problems are of our own making and therefore I need not offer help or advice unless specifically asked because often people need to work through things themselves in their own way. I need to focus more on myself and my own life while being compassionate and loving to those around me without becoming embroiled in their dramas.

I haven't been careful enough with the food I've eaten today and consequently, my bottom is sore from going to the toilet so much and my stomach is not right but otherwise I'm okay. My breast has cooled down – it's still not as cool as the other one and I'm so glad of this two-day break from radiation because of the weekend.

14/4/2019 Sunday

It takes so much energy to stay alive – just to breathe and take yourself from one chair to the other. I've already made the bed and put a load of washing on while John went to the shops but I feel tired and worn out. It's hard to be alive, to keep going, to keep making the effort when you have such small reserves of energy. It makes me think of all those people who have terminal illnesses, are in a lot of pain and are bed ridden. "Life is sweet," John's mum said not long before she died, and added that you would try everything if you knew you were really sick – and I agree. I understand completely why some people travel across the world if they feel there is some hope of relief or a cure. I also understand those who believe that people should never be assisted to die because things can change at any moment. However, those who haven't been through those illnesses haven't got much of a clue even if they're looking after the person with the illness.

To go through major illness yourself opens your eyes to the suffering of many people who are on the brink of life and death and are holding on by a thread. If they have their wits about them and they choose not to eat, they should be allowed not to eat and not be interfered with. Each adult person must take responsibility for their own life and not be pressured into decisions or taking medication they don't want, to prolong a life they don't feel they can continue living.

The radiation machine is enormous – almost as tall as the ceiling with a large disc that is positioned a couple of feet above me as I lie on my back with my arms above my head. It's hard to lie in this position and even these few minutes seem like an eternity as my arms begin to ache. I have to lie perfectly still and I pray each time that it will quickly be over with no side effects or damage to my skin. The machine keeps moving and making strange noises as it shifts and goes into different phases of the process. It's like an alien being searching, detecting, scanning. The whole experience feels futuristic with the screens on the far wall showing my details and a photograph of my bare upper body lying on the table. As the huge disc above my head moves aside, I can see an opening like an eye directly above me. I feel like a person captured by aliens who are carrying out tests on me while I have to lie stock still or be radiation zapped in the wrong spot. I can't feel any pain except in my arms from having them above my head so I try to relax and breathe as normally as possible. The nurses and the radiation therapists are so thoughtful but I can't wait for the end of all this. My life is completely taken over by the treatments. I don't know what other patients do but I just try to get through and be all right for the next day. I haven't got the energy to do much else. I try to do a few jobs around the house but I feel tired and lethargic which forces me to go very slowly. I try to remember that getting through this has to be my priority at the moment as John and my brother and sister keep reminding me.

Joy, who has just phoned, keeps reminding me too. Apart from being a close friend for many years she is a very intuitive person who has really supported me not only through this but also through the death of my brother, Anthony. She also lost a brother some time ago and understands what it has meant to me.

When my dear brother, Anthony, died suddenly in October 2015 the loss my family and I felt couldn't be measured. He died one week after his 55th birthday of a massive stroke. His lovely smile, twinkling eyes and cheery words have been so missed. It's been devastating. After the funeral, the sun was still shining, people around the streets were talking and laughing – everything was going on just as before but how could it, I wondered, when Anthony wasn't there? How could it make any sense? What were we going to do without Anthony's smiling face and light-hearted banter?

There is no doubt that my brother's death has affected me greatly with such excruciating pain sometimes. The world without Anthony in it, Anthony so vital and full of life – it didn't seem possible and has kept gnawing at me for three years. Now I see how damaging to my health all this has been. I feel I can let go of all the sharpest pain of that grief now, and remember Anthony with gratitude for being my brother and a loving presence throughout my life.

15/4/2019 Monday

Another radiation treatment finished! Again, I've come away feeling so lucky. I only need to have nineteen Radiation treatments and I had three months of

Chemotherapy consisting of four treatments, once every three weeks and it has felt and sounded overwhelming at times. But I know that's not much compared with people who are in stages two and three, which means the cancer has spread into the rest of their bodies. Monica, a lady I met in the waiting room, has to have thirty Radiation treatments and had to have twenty nodes removed as the cancer had spread. She showed me the huge red burn across her collar bone from the treatments and said she couldn't sleep last night because of the rubbing of the burnt skin under her arm and how painful and troublesome it was. Brian, another patient who had prostate cancer needed thirty-nine treatments. "We do it for our family," he said, when I said, "Sometimes I feel like, 'that's enough – I don't want to do any more!'" We agreed with Monica that we were scared but we were braving it out. She had the red Chemo drug that I did and I mentioned my allergic reaction to the first drug. She said she'd heard how that could be life-threatening and again I realised what a close shave I'd had. Hopefully now all is easier and I will keep getting better.

It feels like my body has been attacked in every aspect, in every cell, from every angle, in every quarter and it has bravely withstood the attack. When I asked Monica how she first knew about the cancer she said she felt pain under her arm and began to feel around to see what was causing it and discovered a lump and then a couple of lumps and it turned out the cancer had spread to the lymph nodes and she had to have twenty removed. So now I know, a discharge from the nipple, it becoming inverted, pain in the breast or under the arms, lumps, discolouration of the nipple, all need to be investigated immediately when it comes to breast cancer.

16/4/2019 Tuesday

In my imagination I can still do anything but in reality, I have to slow down or stop completely. Sometimes I begin a task such as sweeping the floor and after a few moments I think to myself: "What are you doing? Go and find a chair and sit down!" My body tells me it doesn't have enough energy to do those things that in my mind I think I can do – usually just ordinary things too. Yes, in my imagination I can still do everything and then I look in the mirror and see a dilapidated, depleted old woman looking back at me. I have to take it easy – or so my body keeps reminding me.

17/4/2019 Wednesday

Had my tenth radiation treatment today. I feel fine though rather weary. Last night around 8.30pm I felt three sharp stabs to my right breast. It was very quick and so painful it took my breath away just for a couple of seconds. The stabbing pain was just one at a time over about half an hour but if it had happened any more than that I would have had to go to emergency. Luckily it subsided. I get a bit of prickly pain every now and again throughout the day but nothing too bad. I told the radiation therapists who noted it down and said they could refer me to the nurse but I had already been told what to do before the treatments and they confirmed that would be the advice: a cold pack on the area and two pain killers. They said I would need to contact the clinic if it happened any more frequently though. I feel that I am in good hands with world class specialists, therapists, nurses, and technology – the best of hands actually – not that these machines have hands but they are big and have moving parts and are awe-inspiring.

I saw Brian, the cancer patient, with only six more treatments to go and we had a laugh about the cure killing us rather than the cancer. He admitted that he was scared about having radiation four years ago after surgery and opted not to have it but the cancer returned – I think it was prostate cancer. Everything is scary about all this – the condition and the treatments for both women and men and you have to bring out every bit of bravery you've got, to get through it without being a screaming mess. I think it's best to admit that and move on. We don't want to be weak and wimpy but it is terribly frightening and often painful, uncomfortable and embarrassing as we have to expose private parts of our bodies to complete strangers – albeit medical staff - over prolonged months while you hope and pray that you can get through this with some semblance of dignity and a few more good years of life at the other end.

It confirms to me that it's important to allow ourselves to feel scared and upset but not to let it take over. I asked Monica yesterday whether she had suffered a loss between two and five years ago as I have heard a similar question is asked at one of the cancer retreats and wellness centres. Not surprising to me now, she answered, "Yes, my father." We agreed that getting to the bottom of what causes cancer has been difficult because it's not simply cause and effect – there seem to be many things that come together to cause it because it happens to some people and not to others in similar circumstances. But the "stress" we both agreed has a negative effect on the body, and loss, whether it is connected to a person, a job, a career, a house, investments etc. would cause a huge upheaval in a person's emotional and physical life and I'm thinking this could include spiritual crisis as well.

After the loss of my Mum and my younger brother I know what it means to be in deep grief. To lift yourself out of that and live life in a positive way means not to focus on what you've lost but to focus on all the good things in your life right now. It's easy to let the loss eclipse everything including the present and what you've got now that's good in your life.

18/4/2019 Thursday

Only eight more treatments to go! I'm feeling fine too. My breast is warmer and pinker than the healthy one but, overall, not too bad at all. I can see an end in sight to all this now. I can't wait. Luckily, we've had no visitors because friends and family understand that I just haven't got the energy to deal with them right now but I look forward to when I can see everyone and celebrate. Lack of energy has been a big issue over these last months but feeling really ill has been the worst of all. Hopefully those times are over and soon there will be great and glorious times ahead.

I feel positive today and as though I could dance for sheer happiness. I can't physically do it but I can lift my arms up in the air and I will. The timing of these treatments has been the kindest it could possibly be: I have a four-day break now due to Easter and my right breast is grateful. The timing of everything about this has also been the best it could be – catching the cancer before it spread, having the Chemo through summer so I didn't feel cold in my head from loss of hair, it happening shortly after I put my teaching on hold for a year. I'm grateful and today I feel good.

19/4/2019 Friday

The way I've been feeling during these treatments is that I'm not living, I'm just surviving. I'm wondering when this will change as I wait for the radiation protection cream to dry so I can get dressed. I've washed my hair which is always an ordeal these days and I can't help checking the plug hole every few seconds to see how much of my already diminished hair has fallen out. After the shower I have to dry off completely before I can put the special cream on. Luckily, I can do all these things myself and the cream is helping me considerably. So far, I feel all right after the radiation treatments and I think this is largely due to the cream.

It takes so long in the morning to get ready for the day and to get ready for bed at night that if I don't take care and make a special effort to make the most of it the entire day will go on simply surviving which was par for the course during Chemo but I don't want that to happen now. I'd like there to be at least one thing in the day, and preferably many, that make me happy, that lift my spirit and bring me joy – times when I use my creativity which is a huge part of me and gives me a sense of satisfaction and a feeling of everything being in balance again. I actually feel okay right now.

8.20pm

It looks like I spoke too soon: at around 10.00am this morning I suddenly felt depleted and totally lacking in energy. As I sat at the table, I felt a real weariness and that fatigue has lasted all day.

20/4/2019 Saturday

Have had an upset stomach today but I now know for certain it's the lozenges for the mouth and throat fungus but I need to keep taking them to clear it up.

21/4/2019 Sunday

Easter Sunday has come and gone. It was great to see my sister and all her beautiful family. The kids are not little kids anymore – two of her grandchildren can drive. John and I are now part of the older generation – we're in the grandparent bracket and have been since we became a great aunt and great uncle to Maria's grandchildren. The thing is that I don't feel any different to when I became an aunt to Maria's children. I still feel just as young but of course the mirror reminds me that time has passed and I look different on the outside. But on the inside, I'm still the same young girl I was back then - just the way I'm the same person now even without much hair and looking very much the worse for wear.

25/4/2019 Thursday

I can't seem to move my legs today – they feel stiff and sore and I don't have much energy at all. I suppose it's all part of the radiation side-effects. It's hard to get around or do anything. I'm trying to be patient and not expect too much of myself but I have to keep reminding myself to do that – it doesn't come naturally. I'd like to feel brighter and more energetic and at the moment it seems like it will never happen, but I'm sure to get back at least some of that and I hope that soon I'll be better than ever. I feel breathless too and as though every little task is too much effort.

5.45pm

Today my legs have refused to work properly; they feel wooden and stiff. I feel as though I'm on stilts. My arms and shoulders also feel heavy and tired. I might be Pinocchio with the wooden limbs and the rivets holding them together.

26/4/2019 Friday

Only five more treatments to go! Joy of joys! But I don't want to speak too soon. Today's session went by easily and I hope it'll be the same with all the others. My body's been under continual attack for months now and I'm so looking forward to complete recovery now without being jabbed, prodded, zapped or stretched like I'm on a torture rack.

27/4/2019 Saturday

I'm still battling with this mouth and throat fungus – still taking the tablets otherwise it can quickly get out of hand. I've just remembered, I need to release it – I don't know if I've done it before or maybe I haven't done it properly. I concentrate and relax all the muscles in my throat and mouth – I didn't realise they were so tense – and as I take a deep breath in and then out, I mentally let it go. I'm trying to think of a powerful affirmation to say as I do this: "My mouth and throat are clear and clean, strong and healthy and my tastebuds are better than ever. I rejoice that everything is in perfect health and balance in my whole body, especially my mouth and throat."

28/4/2019 Sunday 5pm

I have had a very bad stomach ache this afternoon. It seemed to come out of nowhere and for three hours I had a fairly horrible time. I drank two cups of hot water and had to lie down on the bed. Yvonne, my dear friend of over forty-eight years, phoned and I think it must have been her prayers and good wishes because now I feel okay again – and I don't have to weigh up if I need to go into emergency. She understands very well what I'm going through as her mother had to go through breast cancer and treatments at different times throughout her life starting in her early thirties – a terrifying thing particularly in the early seventies when the whole of our class at O'Neill College knew things were as serious as they could be. I was scared for Yvonne and her mum though I didn't know any details and I hadn't experienced anything related to cancer then. Throughout this really tough time in my life, Yvonne, who is an artist has sent me a gorgeous homemade card almost every week, often making me laugh with a humorous comment. That sort of support really does ease the pain in a very real way.

8.00pm

Those hours earlier and that pain, mainly in the belly area, reminded me I'm not back to normal yet and things can still change in an instant and not to take anything for granted. I've been going over everything I did, and what I ate and drank to try to pinpoint the cause of all that pain, but I just don't know. I'm so relieved it has settled down. It was actually very scary for a while when I didn't know where it was going and I so much did not want to end up in hospital again. Anyway, the trouble has been averted, thank God.

30/4/2019 Tuesday

The last day of April and I can hardly believe it. I have only three more radiation treatments to go. Today was the first of the last four which are different because the radiation is focussed on the exact spot where the cancer had been and not generally over the entire breast. I have been nervous about these final four treatments because I have been told that they can cause more redness to the area and more irritation but I'm hoping things will flow smoothly and not be a problem.

The machine was set up differently and was very close above me this time. The therapists told me as they were manipulating my position on the table and taking time to get everything exactly right that once it was all set up, the treatment itself would be very quick. It turned out to be exactly one verse, and three quarters of the chorus of "Waltzing Matilda" which I was singing in my head during the whole thing to take my mind off being so nervous.

I saw Doctor Sarah Turner, my radiation specialist too after that. She is marvellous at drawing diagrams and pin pointing exactly how everything works in a way that is easy to understand for a non-medical person like me. She explained how the radiation kills off any microscopic cancer cells that might still exist and be lurking in the breast area and the way it targets the specific area that as recently as the 1980s would have required a mastectomy every time to give the patient the best chance. Now with radiation, mastectomy isn't a foregone conclusion.

She was very happy with the way the treatments were going for me and with the good state of my skin.

I was thrilled to hear it and mentally leapt for joy at the thought that it would soon all be over and the real healing of my body could begin. I asked her what she thought was the best way I could keep healthy and she said that exercising and getting the heart rate up was important, and walking in particular, preferably outdoors, was paramount to good health. Sarah said that's what she does a few times a week and that made me really take note. John has always said, "Don't listen to what a person says but notice what they do." It's the most genuine indicator of what they believe.

1/5/2019 Wednesday

The treatment went well today but I was stretched out on the 'rack' for a bit longer this time. The therapists were apologetic and told me not to worry as they had to make a few adjustments once they were out of the room, so all was in position and ready to go. I couldn't even tell when the radiation started and stopped; all I know is that it took one verse and one chorus of "Waltzing Matilda" in English, one verse and one chorus in French, one verse and one chorus in Italian, one verse in English again and one "God Save the Queen" – to be rounded off with one, God Get Me out of Here!

The therapists finally returned and said it was all finished, so that was a relief. I have a few more texta dots on my breast as well like a living road map to direct them. They are all so kind and careful and precise. They always talk to me a little at the beginning before they have to concentrate hard and usually ask me what I'll be doing that day and what I have planned. I've been running out of things to say. They're young and vital and I don't want to say, "I'm just trying to survive at the moment and even this bit of cheeriness and conversation on my part is a huge effort for me," instead I try to think of something interesting that's also true so I briefly mention that next year I'm having three children's books published and they are surprised and happy for me. I'm just about to cheekily say to them, "When the books are on the shelves for sale next year you can boast that not only have you met the author but you've met her boobs as well!" but another therapist comes in at that very moment and I miss my opportunity as they get caught up in rechecking an important positioning of the right side of my body.

6.05pm

John and I are having our tea and I am sitting at the table when I suddenly feel something on my left shin. There is a spreading pain and I know instantly that something is wrong. "What's the matter with me?" I say anxiously as I lift up my trouser leg to have a look at the area. To my shock I see a big, purple bruise about two inches in diameter. It has appeared in an instant out of nowhere. It is also raised in a bump and very painful. I know for certain I have not knocked my leg anywhere and no accident has happened to cause this and that's why I begin to panic.

John looks at it closely and admits it's very odd though he remains calm. We both agree I will have to be taken in to emergency. It hurts terribly and looks bad. The suddenness of this has really shocked me and my breathing is fast and shallow although I'm trying to keep calm. I need to pack a few things in case I have to stay in hospital – it's no good putting the pressure on John later - I have to be prepared. I'm scared it might be a blood clot or that other bruises may spring up.

We debate whether to call an ambulance and when John says he wants to drive me in I'm grateful and relieved. We get into the car and drive to Cabrini Hospital and luckily within thirty-five minutes or so we are there. I see a truly kind doctor, Ian Walton, and he is not overly concerned about it and can't say exactly what has caused it, but it's a possibility that the Chemotherapy and continuing radiation have something to do with it. He does an ultrasound which shows it isn't a blood clot. After examining me and making sure there are no other bruises, he says I can go home and the relief I feel is indescribable.

I don't want anything interfering with my last two radiation treatments. I almost feel desperate to get it finished now. He assures me that if no other bruises appear, I should be all right. He is confident and John has told me he felt it would be all right too so I feel happy and relieved and extremely tired so we head home immediately after thanking the doctor a few times.

Four hours later we are back home and I am congratulating myself on my good luck that things have worked out well after a very scary start to the evening. Of course, I could have been a lot luckier and not have had it happen at all – but still, I didn't have to stay in hospital, so I take a big, grateful breath and settle down to snooze in front of the television.

2/5/2019 Thursday

Two verses and two choruses of "Waltzing Matilda" today – it was much quicker than yesterday.

3/5/2019 Friday 7.45pm

I have felt nauseous all day today. I have been nervous too and I think these treatments magnify any feelings of illness or discomfort. But all that aside – I have finished all my Radiation Treatment – all nineteen treatments! And Chemo is over. I have rung the bell in the corridor with three resounding rings – one for good health, one for happiness and one for hope that the cancer never returns – that's what they meant to me, and they were joyful rings which made me feel emotional as any lovely sound does. Christine, the nurse was with me and she then led me to the huge painting of a tree I had noticed along the corridor from the beginning. I didn't realise it was decorated by the patients and was a work in progress, and now it was my turn to choose a colour, dip my finger in the paint and add a dot around the tree which represents a leaf. I chose pink, the colour of love and placed my dot high up in the sky for peace, love and hope. Then the nurse explained about taking it easy over the next couple of weeks as the side-effects relating to radiation such as possible skin burn would peak then. After that I handed over the chocolates and card I had prepared for all the staff to share as my thank you for all their hard work and dedication.

The final treatment took two verses and one-and-three-quarter choruses of the old standby, "Waltzing Matilda" so it was quick and efficient – as usual. I felt happy and a bit teary as I left, but mostly I felt incredibly lucky.

In the waiting room, before this treatment session, I had spoken to another patient, Sheryl, who had been diagnosed with third stage breast cancer so she was to have thirty sessions. Again, she admitted how surprised she was about her diagnosis and how she hadn't felt any pain. Her cancer was discovered through the two-yearly mammogram. I was seeing clearer than ever that although none of the women I had spoken to felt any physical pain they had experienced deep emotional pain: in the past recent years Sheryl had mourned the death of her mother and the loss of her marriage. Her advice to me was to keep away from negative people and not to listen to people's stories about others they had heard of or knew who had had breast cancer as it was all negative and usually misleading which I had discovered along the way as well. Sheryl said her husband was a good man but he was too hard to live with as nothing was ever good enough for him and she was a very positive person while he was very negative. They had tried many times to reconcile but now, finally, it was over.

In my heart I felt truly grateful for having such a wonderful husband and again I couldn't believe how lucky I had been to have had the cancer diagnosed so soon – before it had completely taken hold. As it is, the medications have completely ravaged my body, but I know it is ready to bounce back again given half a chance. And I have a firm resolve to help it all I can.

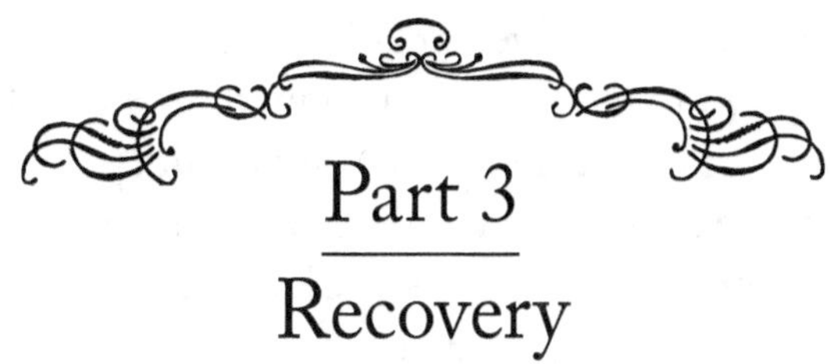

Part 3

Recovery

4/5/2019 Saturday

I've felt sick all day with an upset stomach and nausea. My breast is okay but very tender, pink and warm - which is only to be expected.

5/5/2019 Sunday

I know it's important for me to move out of the past and to live my life more in the present. I am grateful for the past and all the help I've received and now I want to be able to step forward and bring only the good things with me and leave behind all that hasn't worked. I want to be able to go forward happily with hope and trust that all will be well without feeling guilty for being happy. I've had enough of being nervous and fearful and not being able to relax and enjoy all the good that comes my way. When I was at secondary school in the seventies many girls didn't go on to further studies and many were not encouraged by their families to follow successful careers. The expectation was to get married and have a family. I was going against the accepted pattern in my family background by wanting to be a teacher, but Dad supported me wholeheartedly and Mum was okay with it too although she hoped at any moment that I would wake up and stop studying so much. A large part of my career centred on teaching secondary school boys – hard to believe due to my shyness but I found I was fine with children of all ages - even ones in their teens. One thing Anthony said to me which was something he had learnt as a singer and performer was, "Own your space – you're alive – you're meant to have it. Stretch out your arms. All that space around you is yours. Claim it! You don't have to be scared or meek or apologetic about it. Just realise you're entitled to it."

6/5/2019 Monday

A breast cancer magazine arrived in the post today filled with articles about the latest treatments and research, schemes to raise money for them, and people's personal stories of their experiences. One is about a young mother living with the threat of breast cancer that has metastasised which means it has spread into other areas of her body. It is described as "Triple Negative" cancer, "one of the most aggressive forms of breast cancer which doesn't respond to the easier treatments using tablets." It confirms for me that this type of cancer is one of the deadliest and worst in terms of it spreading quickly and silently.

Again, I can't help feeling incredibly grateful for the fact that I didn't get it at a young age and haven't had to deal with young children as well. It's been hard enough to get through the Surgery, Chemo and Radiation with just me to think of. The article highlights how this beautiful mother is accepting her shortened life span with "gratitude and grace".

7/5/2019 Tuesday

I still have this mouth and throat fungal infection that I'm coping with. It takes away the pleasure of eating: a good part of that is the aftertaste of foods when you finish the meal and you can still taste and enjoy the delicious flavours for a good while afterwards. It's a feeling of contentment and that all's well with the world, but instead there is always a bitter aftertaste now and a slightly unsettled feeling in the stomach which can easily become nausea or indigestion or just a general sense of being unwell. Still, all this is better than it was while I was on Chemo. Then it was horrendous – now it's just unpleasant and annoying.

12/5/2019 Sunday

An article in the Herald/Sun: "Cancer Test Hope" tells of a new blood test to detect breast cancer which will eventually do away with mammograms. This will be one of the big changes which will improve the lot of all women, as now one in eight Australian women is diagnosed with breast cancer in their lifetime. This test could save so much hassle, worry and pain. We are moving closer all the time to doing away with Chemo and Radiation.

It feels like my body has been through a complete devastation and it's lucky to still be functioning. I am sincerely grateful to be alive and I intend to make the most of this second chance. My body is already making a comeback: my hair is getting thicker and the bald patches have fuzz growing in them which gets fuzzier each day and not one hair is falling out – every single hair seems to be clinging on stronger and bolder than ever before.

One main thing I've learnt throughout this experience which I've mentioned before and which has surprised me is the immense respect that is owed to my resilient body for the way it keeps bouncing back, striving always to be well, to recover and to improve. It has truly been an inspiration to me and is due much more attention, care and respect than I have ever given it. There have been times throughout these last months when I've felt I couldn't go on but my body has led the way and shown that it would go on – that there are unexpected and hidden wells of strength to draw on that will get us through the most devastating and terrifying experiences. From now on I want to make sure that I always treat myself well and give my body the full respect it deserves.

17/5/2019 Friday 1.36pm

Today is officially my last day of treatment – of all treatments, both Chemo and Radiation – and I can't believe the day has finally come. I count this as the last day because I was told that the side-effects would peak for up to two weeks after the final physical dose of radiation, and that symptoms would likely worsen up till that point. I should be jumping up and down for joy but firstly, I don't have the energy and secondly, I've had three pretty shaky days. I'm okay in the morning but by the afternoon I've been feeling a stomach ache coming on and it continues into the evening and last night it went till 10pm with so much pain and cramping I thought I would have to go back into emergency. It's been horrible and I don't know what's causing it. I was getting this symptom at the beginning of the Radiation treatments and John has reminded me that this was happening during Chemo too but I had forgotten. The pain extends right across under the breasts and sometimes spreads lower to the abdomen – it's brutal. The whole region from below the belly button to just under the breasts is bad but the pain moves up and down that area. Today I have to get to the bottom of it and find out if a certain food or drink is triggering it so I can stop it from ever happening again.

I've been tentative about everything today, afraid that it will start up again. It just shows that as soon I think I'm returning to normal I'm quickly reminded that I'm not and that I still need to be careful about everything. I'm feeling very tired and sleepy now so I need to have a proper rest in bed. It's so easy to take for granted how good it is to be able to eat and drink. I had already started to forget about the difficulties of all that and how debilitating and unhappy the situation is when you are forced to watch every mouthful you eat and drink and it must be of the very plainest sort.

I still feel a bit frightened of any other bruises appearing and of the "stomach" ache returning – hopefully it's the last of both things.

19/5/2019 Sunday

My legs have not been comfortable since I started Radiation treatment. It's a strange thing but it has affected them: they don't feel right and they sometimes twitch and move when I'm trying to sit and rest. Sometimes it feels like the blood isn't flowing smoothly – it's like singing "sausages" and not "spaghetti" as our Grade 6 singing teacher, Mrs Shepherd, used to say and she'd show us with her hand using her thumb and forefinger – smooth like a stick of spaghetti, not staccato like sausages. That's how it feels in my legs occasionally: that the flow is being blocked and the veins are like a string of sausages, separate and bumpy, stopping the blood from flowing smoothly. On the back of my left hand where the Chemo was injected intravenously over many hours, one of the veins is now like that – a little bit of it must have collapsed because it didn't look like that beforehand.

The treatments have finished and I almost am too! One slightly better thing is I've read in the Radiation Therapy Booklet that cramps are a side-effect of radiation. I have never wanted to read these books or be too focussed on side-effects and illness but I was feeling so sick that I thought it couldn't make me feel any worse and actually it did explain what was happening to me. Radiation can affect the lining of the stomach, no matter where it is given, making it more sensitive and prone to cramps.

23/5/2019

My head is almost all covered in hair again now – except for one small bald patch. It's dark brown, very short, fuzzy sort of hair, quite soft to the touch, with wisps of some longer hair at the back and sides, particularly on one side. Maybe a new me is emerging. I hope so! A more self-assured me – a more poised me who can deal with people in a mature, adult way instead of getting flustered and self-conscious.

24/5/2019 Friday

Somehow I need to start again. I don't want to fall into the same traps as before I got ill. I want to be as happy as I can be but I don't know what to do to change those patterns that interfere with this. Maybe it's about choosing what I enjoy and leaving out the rest – but I don't think I know how to do that. My focus has always been on looking after others. I have spent the last forty years doing that including a big block of eight years taking care of Mum after she had a massive stroke which left her incapacitated and unable to live alone. But that's been over for years now and I'm still churning over past events and wrong decisions I feel I've made. What am I going to do to change this? What am I going to do for myself? What do I actually want to happen in my life? What steps do I need to take to make that happen?

31/5/2019 Friday

After a week of trying to do a bit more movement and meditation I feel more peaceful about everything. The weather is cold which has been helping my breast quite a bit. I've noticed that throughout the Radiation treatments and aftermath my breast is hotter to the touch than the healthy one. I've been very glad of the cold weather. Everything in my body is settling down and I'm feeling a bit more like myself. My stomach is still sensitive but I can feel improvements happening.

1/6/2019 Saturday

It's hard to believe that we are halfway through the year. Today John and I went to Emerald – a 25 minute drive which was great. We had lunch at the bakery café` there and I had a mild curry pie which was a mistake – it was a bit too hot and my body wasn't ready for it. After I ate it, I had to rush to the toilet about five times.

Sometimes I think I'm almost back to normal and then I'm quickly reminded that I'm not all right yet. Be patient! Slow down! seems to be my body's constant message. I'll try not to ignore it. I know it's not worth it as I've ended up having an uncomfortable afternoon through my own silly decision. Plain foods are still the safest for me and I have to be careful about what I eat and drink as both my stomach and throat are very sensitive.

I feel happy though because we had a pleasant drive and even though it was a showery day it was really enjoyable and we were able to do something different as well as being away from the house.

8/6/2019 Saturday

Today I've actually had a cup of tea and two biscuits. This is the first time I've enjoyed this since I started Chemo on the 17th of December last year. So things do come back after Chemo – and this is proof positive! I used to love tea and biscuits and coffee and cake but haven't been able to stand the sight of them for all these past months – maybe now is the beginning of getting my taste back. What a great day this is!

This whole process has been utterly debilitating, draining and revolting. It has left me feeling and looking like a 90-year-old – but having said that, I'm still alive and with prospects of a good future with maybe many years to come.

13/6/2019 Thursday

I look forward to some happy get-togethers after all this is over. The people I care about – both family and friends, I really cherish – and I have good reason to for they are all beautiful, unselfish souls. To be supportive without being overbearing is a fine line to tread and they have proved that it can be done.

"Prison, illness and need, reveal the heart of a friend". It's another one of those old Italian proverbs - one my Mum used to quote and it rings so true. It's under extreme circumstances that many things become as clear as crystal. When I think of all the help that I've received over these last eight months, I can feel tears springing to my eyes immediately. Many people prayed for me, some sent me cards, flowers and gifts, others left things at the door for me, some sent texts, emails and the occasional phone call which was quick when they could hear I was struggling with my voice. My family was magnificent – they kept away, which is what I asked for. My brother, Vincent and sister-in-law, Lorrie, phoned daily from Queensland and I saw my sister, Maria, every day and apart from that John was my mainstay. I think about all those friends and family one by one and how lovely they are and I thank them all sincerely in my heart. How lucky I've been!

Despite all this it has been a horrific time, but it has highlighted who really cares and has revealed the kindness in their hearts because even when they wanted to come and see me, they respected my wishes and let me be. I wasn't up to having visitors – I simply didn't have enough energy to cope with conversations. It was just good to know that friends and family were supporting me without being physically here. They were doing everything they could for me, offering their help, asking if I wanted a visit and respecting my feelings – not forcing themselves on me or being in my face or wanting to see how I was, out of curiosity. To keep away and not call too often showed real caring to me because that's what I had asked for and everyone knew I was being taken good care of by John and my sister so they could physically step back. All their enquiries, cards, gifts and good wishes meant the world to me because through the very worst of it I knew I was truly loved, supported and cared for.

17/6/2019 Monday

My hair is growing back very strangely. I noticed a week or two ago that the hair on my legs was growing back hairier than ever and in a really hard stubble. Luckily that has softened now as it has lengthened. It's been the same under my arms. My head is turning into a rough carpet, thickly matted and different lengths. It had completely stopped growing for three months and continued to fall out so my head was bald and patchy. Now it's almost completely covered in a thick mat of hair but it looks and feels weird – not like my hair at all. It is becoming incredibly thick – as though it is making up for lost time with a wild tangle of rampaging undergrowth. Having no hair was no good but having too much is equally alarming.

I wonder how long it will take for my body to get back into balance. I know it's trying very hard – my poor, old decimated body. Everything about cancer is pretty scary. Sheryl and I agreed about this in the Radiation waiting room. But I said that I had from the very beginning decided to – in my own words, "brave it out" and I would continue to stick to my original intention. She smiled and agreed that was what we all had to do otherwise things were worse. I could see all the people going through that clinic were scared but brave, as are so many other women at the shops, in their cars, on public transport, everywhere around, as I realise more and more how common breast cancer is and how many thousands are coping with it at any given moment. And it makes me more determined than ever to withstand, to endure, to be as brave as I can be and not let fear take hold.

18/6/2019 Tuesday

Haven't felt any good today. I have felt that same tightness at the top of my stomach and under my breasts right across my torso and a general feeling of not being well. I shouldn't have eaten because it made me feel worse. It's been painful all afternoon and now it's 8.15pm and I'm still struggling. This is the same as what used to happen sometimes after having radiation.

Every time I think it's all behind me, I'm reminded that it isn't over and that I need to be more aware and more careful about everything I eat and drink. This has been a tough day to get through.

20/6/2019 Thursday

What a crazy time this has been full of so much physical pain and discomfort. There's been no time for fear or anxiety in the full-on work of trying to cope in just getting through each day. It's been a horrendous experience but I'm still here to talk about it so I'm one of the very lucky ones. I did feel fear once – when the instantaneous bruise appeared on my leg while I was sitting at the table. I felt vulnerable and as though everything could spin quickly out of control – if it could happen so suddenly out of nowhere, it could happen again, and all over the body including the brain. Because of its suddenness, it's been the most frightening – all the other symptoms, side-effects, aches and pains have just been a dull round of things to endure and pray hard that they would hurry up and pass.

LIFE LESSON: BE PATIENT

After such a massive assault on the body by the cancer itself and the treatments, it takes time to get better. Be patient with yourself and with the process of healing.

21/6/2019 Friday

Feeling very flat this morning – not much energy – and finding it hard to get going.

22/6/2019 Saturday

I'm feeling a very noticeable hotness in one area of my right shin. I'm scared it could be leading to another one of those instant bruises but I'm keeping that to myself as I don't want to worry John, especially when I'm hoping it may be nothing and it will pass. I've felt it three or four times today and have looked down in apprehension to check my leg but luckily, it's fine. I'm really wary since the last time it happened so suddenly without any warning. I try to be aware of my whole body and how

I'm feeling so I can isolate what effects any given food or drink or medication has on me and whether something uncomfortable or painful is either minor or serious, that way I keep a close check on everything and prevent problems. This is also why I avoid painkillers: I want to know what's going on and what's causing the discomfort so I can stop it at the source. I don't want to merely mask the problem. I can put up with a certain amount of pain or discomfort and I know I've got the painkillers to fall back on.

I do know that I'm getting stronger each day but I also know it's not a straight line forward as sometimes the recovery seems to take a few steps back. I've discovered that if I'm careful not to eat or drink anything too hot or too cold I can avoid a huge amount of pain. It stops the severe cramping in my stomach and my whole torso area which can last for hours and hours. No food or drink is worth that discomfort, especially now that I know what causes it and how I can avoid it. Even all these weeks after the end of the treatments I need to be very careful or I suffer unnecessarily. I have also discovered that I need to eat good food and not too much of it – mainly vegetables and fruit with very small amounts of meat or fish. I can have chocolate and sweets now but not cream – it gives me an upset stomach straight away and results in many trips to the toilet. I'm glad I have found this out so I can manage better.

23/6/2019 Sunday

John and I had a drive to Mornington today and from there drove to Hastings after that. It was a great day with perfect weather – sunny and warm enough without a jacket and the sea looked magnificent. We actually had lunch at the King's Creek Hotel and the food was very tasty.

Now back at home at 4.00pm I have a really bad stomach ache. It's this sort of thing that reminds me to take more care. The bread and butter pudding for dessert was delicious but a bit too hot for me. I should have waited longer for it to cool down. What an idiot I was! And now because of my greediness and impatience who knows how long this stomach ache will last! I'm very annoyed with myself because I could have avoided this pain and discomfort – no food is worth it, no matter how delicious it is.

7.35pm

As it turned out, the pain lasted only two hours this time which was much shorter than in the past, but I've made up my mind not to let it happen again.

30/6/2019 Sunday 2.15pm

Exactly half way through the year. My hair is now greyish and short – close to my head. It has never been this short except after I was born, 61 years ago. The most unpleasant thing about it is that it feels breezy all over my head and around my neck and ears and because it's winter it makes me feel very cold. I still prefer this to the heat and the horrible hotness of the Chemo and Radiation treatments. I've taken to wearing hats and beanies but they quickly seem to make my head feel hot and uncomfortable.

My tongue and throat are still a concern and I'm sucking on an anti-fungal lozenge right now. John has assured me this fungal infection will eventually pass as my body gets stronger so I feel confident too, especially as John's been through serious medical problems and seen his way through them.

I think our faeces is a good indicator of whether we're well or not and I'm pleased that mine is looking more normal now – although it still looks strange, it actually looks something like poo and not a gelatinous mass without shape, as it has been over the last months. Before the Chemo I would never have imagined that looking at poo could be so traumatic.

8.00pm

I've just had the biggest vomit I've ever had since I was a little child. I kept heaving and luckily, I made it to the toilet or the mess would have been disgusting. I think it was for the best even though it was a ghastly experience because the pain was becoming really severe right across under my breasts including the top of my stomach. I had some pizza for lunch. I don't know exactly what caused the cramping an hour and a half later – whether it was the pizza or the glass of cold water I had with it which was a bit too cold, or the anti-fungal lozenge I had after that. Maybe it was a combination of things. When I had a dose of antacid, on John's suggestion, just before I vomited, I thought it was a brilliant idea which hadn't occurred to me. And I think ultimately it *was* because it emptied out my stomach completely and now I finally feel relief from the cramping pains although the whole area is still sore to the touch.

I didn't know my stomach could hold such a huge amount of watery substance. I still feel a pain high up in my gut. I hope it's over – it's exhausting and nauseating as well as painful and scary. This continues to remind me that I need to be extra careful about everything.

1/7/2019 Monday

Feeling tender and sore around the upper stomach area this morning and generally low in energy. I want to be well and I'm determined to be well but my body keeps reminding me that I'm not all right yet and that I need to be more patient.

2/7/2019 Tuesday

Still feeling unwell – low in energy and not good around the top of the stomach and the area right across under my breasts – quite painful but in a dull ache sort of way – I'm hoping that's because it's passing and I'll soon feel well.

4/7/2019 Thursday

I'm feeling better today than I've felt for a few days and have done some cooking – barley soup and a stew. I'm getting back into things but I don't necessarily want things to be the same as they were before anyway. I want to fully regain my strength and be able to do all the cooking again as my sister has helped a lot over these past months and it's time for her to be relieved of that responsibility.

I'm sure most people would say, "You're over sixty; you've lived your life; you've had your career; you can bow out now – step back and let the younger ones have a go"

– and I do let the younger ones have a go. I encourage them to develop their talents and pursue their goals as I always have and actually help them to fulfil their dreams if I can. As a teacher, I've made that a large part of my life's work. I want them to have as many opportunities as there are to have and I would never take somebody else's chance away from them. Luckily, I can see all the young people in my life pursuing their studies, work, careers, interests, and everything else they want to do to have happy lives.

Many people think it's too late as a senior to dream of a new career or a new direction in life, but I don't agree. I still feel I have things to do and I have always had a passion for children's literature and a desire to get things published. I have always written stories, poems and songs ever since I can remember just because I loved making them up even if no one else saw them and even if I had no time to devote to it because of work and family: teaching takes up almost everything and my parents always needed a lot of help. It didn't stop me writing – nothing ever did. Since I began teaching part-time a few years ago, I was able to devote a bit more of my energy towards it and two years ago three of my children's books were accepted by a publisher.

This is a dream finally come true for me and the fulfilment of a life-long passion that I've never had enough time for. Now I want to bring it to the fore and pursue it fully. I don't have the energy I once had and I feel worn out at the moment but I think my body will make a come-back and I will be encouraging it all the way, just as much as I've encouraged others in the past. I want to see if I can get things published so that children and maybe adults too can enjoy the things I've written as much as I've enjoyed writing them. I really believe it's never too late to fulfil your dreams, to change course, to try something different, to put your time and energy into something else – it's not too late while you're still alive because inside I think most of us are children. We might look different on the outside with our wrinkles and grey hair but I can say for myself, I still feel young on the inside.

I still have the hope of fulfilling one of my dreams; I have aspirations to be a published author - not just a writer; I still passionately want to share my stories with others, and now that I've been through the last eight months of serious, debilitating illness I know that nothing will dampen this desire – if breast cancer didn't do it, I don't think anything will. My desire is just as strong as it was when I didn't have time to pursue it and still did. So now I'm going to follow it to where it leads me and if it means only three books get published then that will be good enough, but I will certainly try for more. The flame of creativity is just as alive in me as it ever was and burning brightly and I won't keep it hidden any more.

20/7/2019 Saturday

This week I saw my G.P. and also my Radiation specialist for the first time after my treatment ended. Both were happy with my progress. The specialist, Sarah, said my skin looked the best she had seen on any patient in a long time. She gave me a thorough examination and noted that my right breast was still warmer to the touch than the left one. So, I'm still cooking away with the radiation almost two months after the treatments are over. The good thing is, I can't feel it and I actually feel pretty good. The bad thing is, I overdid it and have had a bit of a setback. My mouth and tongue have been worse and my gut has been very unhappy, giving me aches and pains and indigestion – this was because we ate out to celebrate the good news and it's also a reaction against the nervousness I felt on the two days about seeing the doctors and finding out what they had to report about the results. Every bit of stress, tension and nervousness plays havoc with my body now. Every emotion seems amplified as does the effect it has on me.

I was so relieved it was all good news because the truth is that I was worried about any lumps that might have reappeared. I think this fear is simply to be expected given the circumstances – it's a disease that seems to creep in silently like "Fog", the poem by Carl Sandburg we studied in Grade 6, but unlike the enigmatic fog in the poem, cancer is insidious and deadly.

I've been feeling like I did about a month ago and John has reminded me that recovery is not a linear process – there are usually upsets and reverses and the road to recovery is not a straight path but is often full of bumps and backtracking.

21/7/2019 Sunday

I'm still dealing with the fungal mouth and throat problem. It's not as bad as it was months ago but it's still there. I think it's an indication of how well I am – I'm better than I was but with a way to go in overall wellness. It might be the reason plaque seems to build up so quickly between my teeth. My stomach and gut are also still a problem with constant pains and the threat of nausea and vomiting. I'm not complaining, as I'm much better than I was even two months ago let alone six months ago.

I have a really strong sense of how short life is so I want to get well as quickly as I can and in the meantime enjoy every day I've got. I don't want to overdo it though. After my wonderful brother, Anthony, died I came to the conclusion that waiting for the right moment to do the things you want to do will probably mean you never get to do them.

I thought there would still be time for us to review our fun children's show, "The Beach Ball Band", which we'd created, worked on together and performed in over thirty venues around Victoria about twenty years ago, my husband, my brother and I, but there turned out to be no more time because no matter how long I live, Anthony is gone. The people you love may not be around even if you are. I didn't think everything would be cut short like that. I probably should have known because growing up in the sixties and seventies, my brothers and I had creative talents but it seemed we had no way of developing them – we were blocked at every turn and over the years the frustration was immense – even up till now. We weren't encouraged to develop our creativity. It wasn't understood that we could make a living out of singing and dancing and writing. They were considered hobbies by most people not just our parents. My sister had no chance at all as she was married at seventeen and fulfilling all the expectations by having a baby at eighteen.

Now that I've been going through this experience of my own illness, I'm doubly aware of the shortness of life and how quickly everything can change. In a breath you can be taken in a completely different direction and without good health you can't do much – it's hard even to get through the day. Illness forces you into being a survivor and makes you put all your energy into recovery. I've been there and I'm starting to find my way out of it. As my body gets stronger, I've been putting more time into the things that bring me a lot of happiness, and that means making up poems and stories and songs. In 2017 I signed the contract with Big Sky Publishing, an Australian company for my three children's books. A dream came true for me that day which has had this craziness in the middle of it. But that's all right - I won't give up. Instead of this year, as originally intended, they will be released next year and while the illustrator, Nancy Bevington, is still working on them, the covers, summaries and blurbs will be displayed at a worldwide Book Fair next month where publishers display what's coming up for sale. That spurs me on to be hopeful and to create more and to spend more time on the things I love doing.

There are big patches of real happiness now despite the tummy tantrums and the lack of energy and the mouth worries. My body has shown me that it can get through this, that I can be well and that one day I can put this behind me. I trust in the process of recovery even if it isn't a straight line ahead.

22/7/2019 Monday

I can hardly believe it, but in the last few days, I've noticed that my eyebrow colour has come back – my natural auburn colour which had turned to grey overnight has now returned to normal. It's amazing! So, it's true that things will come back. Although I was always hopeful, I hadn't really believed it.

23/7/2019 Tuesday

What can I say to you that would be of any help? Courage! Perseverance! This is going to call on everything you've got. Don't wimp out on yourself. Be brave! You'll get through. Call on all the help you can get. You can have a party afterwards to celebrate and thank everyone. Keep going! Keep going! Even when you feel you want to give up – keep going! Things will change. Things will get better. Even at those terrible times when you feel that it's too hard and maybe life isn't worth living. It won't always be this bad. Unforeseen things might happen, that's true but that's in the future and we can't know about that. Say to yourself: "This moment I can endure it – this moment. Only this moment exists and in this moment I'm okay." And for me personally, there's someone who truly cares about me right now so I need to keep going. I'm looking forward to having a clear head, to smelling the freesias again in spring, to seeing the lilacs bloom in my front yard, to being well enough to walk around the lakes and see the sunrise at Frog Hollow Reserve.

28/7/2019 Sunday

I've had a terrible fright today. John was feeling sick

when he got up. He had been awake since 4.00am not feeling well and he struggled through many hours while I was asleep and unaware. His heart has been out of sync. He has been suffering from Arrhythmia for the last few years and this happens on and off. His skin felt cold and clammy and he had a pain under his ribs. His temperature was 34.6 – too low but he didn't want to go into hospital; he wanted to wait and see if it would clear up and right itself again. I try to respect his decisions about his health while telling him what I feel would be best. We don't want to panic about it because we've been managing serious problems for a long time going back to when I looked after my mum for years after she had that major, life-changing stroke. We have had to learn to weigh things up or we'd be in hospital every week about something.

3.00pm

Thank God it has all come good and John feels fine. He doesn't want to see the doctor about it and says he feels well again. I continue to hope and pray.

1/8/2019 – 31/8/2019

A month of steadily getting better but also of ups and downs. I'm loving the coolness of winter. I don't mind how cold it gets after all the hotness of the Chemo. I don't miss the flurry of hair falling over my face and pillow every night either. It was a horrible feeling throughout those first three months. Now my hair is springy and wiry with hard, tight curls at the back and looking like it was always black. It's weird for me as I've always had light-coloured hair but it's better than not having any.

I didn't think hair would be much of an issue for me but it has been and I understand the worry surrounding it now. Apart from keeping our heads warm and comfortable, our hair is a big part of our identity. When we suddenly look different it can throw us off balance and those close to us as well, as we try to readjust to the suddenly different appearance. Sometimes we want to say, "Yes it's still me under this bald head – or under this unruly mop of hair."

For the last few days I've had a light headache that hasn't lifted and a slight heaviness above the eyes and at times I've felt my pulse beating in my head. I had my blood pressure checked at the chemist, three days in a row and it was higher than usual – around 160/85.

I'll have to see my G.P. as this can't be ignored. I know enough about blood pressure and headaches to realise it can be dangerous. My Dad, Mum and younger brother all died of strokes and my brother had just turned 55 that week, so I have to pay attention to this and follow it up. If I must die, I want to die healthy – not like my dear Mum who was incapacitated for all those long years before she died. And my father who kept having small strokes which his specialist called "stutter strokes" for years before a really horrible one carried him off.

3/9/2019 Tuesday

Blood pressure was 170/90 when I visited the clinic to have it checked so Doctor Frankel said he'd be happier if I went onto blood pressure medication. He knows how much I'd rather not be on any tablets but I agreed it was a good idea as my pressure has been elevated for quite a few days now. I have to accept I'm sixty-one, not thirty-one and that I've been lucky not to have been on medication before now.

I was feeling more like my normal self today and the doctor said I was looking better than last time. He said my hair would settle down as I pointed out that it was thickening up but growing strangely – so that's something to look forward to, although I'm grateful to have any hair, strange or not. It looks like I've tried to blow dry it and done a bad job of it as it's all springy and puffy as though my scalp is covered in hundreds of cow licks. If I pat it down that's what it feels like and it won't stay down - just like me!

On our way home I felt relieved that everything was in hand and that, as usual, Doctor Frankel had done an excellent job in diagnosing and dispensing treatments with accuracy and care. He is a great doctor.

4/9/2019 Wednesday

It's incredible what difference a quarter of a tablet can make! My blood pressure today is 139/78 and my pulse rate is 73 after taking a quarter of a tablet yesterday and a quarter this morning. This is good cause for celebration: we are invited for lunch at Maria's place. What could be better!

26/9/2019 Thursday

This morning has been the easiest so far with regard to the toilet, showing me that my insides have improved in a major way. I know health issues go backwards and forwards and the road to recovery is not a straight path but this is a huge red-letter day for me. And speaking of red - I'm glad to say I don't feel revulsion at the sight of certain shades of red anymore.

My hair is still strange and springy and has grown into a colour it never was in all my life – browny black – instead of the auburn it always has been. As John says, "Your hair has come back – we just don't know whose hair it is!"

2/10/2019 Wednesday

It was during this month exactly one year ago that this journey began. I was getting some acupuncture done by Lee, a highly recommended specialist in the field who is extremely intuitive as well as skilful. It turned out to be completely different to what I expected. I was going for physical health – I was experiencing arthritis in my knee and hands and thought it might be beneficial without having to take medication and it ended up helping me in a completely different way. I was still holding onto a lot of grief over my brother – during one of the sessions I was a bit emotional about one of the songs playing in the background as it was one Anthony used to sing. I didn't cry but I felt that I easily could. Next time, Lee, put one of the only three needles he uses, at the side of my right wrist without telling me why he had changed its position since the last visit.

During that week I listened to my brother's CD with great joy for the very first time since he had gone and I was able to listen to it happily every day that week. I still felt sad but that sharp, jagged edge to the pain was gone. And every time I thought about Anthony, I remembered a joke he used to tell or something funny he'd often say, and the instant tears that would spring to my eyes were mixed with a chuckle or laughter instead of the choking lump I always felt in my throat and the pain

I'd feel in my chest with every memory of him.

At the beginning of the next acupuncture session, Lee told me he was treating me for the releasing of grief and had started this treatment the previous week. I didn't know acupuncture could be used for that so I can say with one hundred per cent certainty that it works. I had no idea what Lee had done but I had experienced its amazing effect. After that I had another three sessions and felt better and more peaceful each time about Anthony's passing. It was as though something heavy on my heart had lifted and a blockage had been removed.

It was after one of those sessions that I had a discharge out of my right breast. It was such a small amount that at first I didn't notice. Only after a few days did I see the little brownish yellow spots on my crop top and realised this liquid hadn't been moisture left after my showers but something that was oozing out of my nipple. I didn't think much of it but when I showed John, he was concerned about it and said I needed to have it checked out by the doctor straight away. So the day before my next acupuncture session, I cancelled it and booked an appointment to see Doctor Frankel.

The mammogram he sent me to have, showed there was something to investigate and from there began a year-long experience which has surprised and shocked me. Both the doctor and surgeon said the discharge had nothing to do with the breast cancer which was detected in the ultrasound and then the biopsy I was given. This seemed very odd to me as, ironically, it was that which started the investigation, otherwise I would have waited for my two-yearly mammogram to come around which would have been in September of this year. By that time the cancer would certainly have spread, and being the type that it was, it would have been a very different outcome for me.

I really believe that the acupuncture helped to release something destructive which the grief had blocked up or it was the grief itself which was quietly destroying me or maybe it was neither of those things and I'm right off the mark. Whatever it was, the discharge led to the cancer being discovered and for my life to be saved and early enough for me to be able to make a full recovery. If that's not called miraculous, I don't know what is.

8.10pm

For the last 24 hours my breast has been giving me trouble. It started last night with the stabbing pains but it didn't subside after a few minutes, it went on and under my arm has been sore too. I don't like to admit it but I've been trying to feel around because I can't help being a bit worried that there might be a lump. And that is exactly what's so horrible about having had cancer – you can't ever fully get away from it. The thought that it could come back lurks at the back of your mind and comes to the fore when you don't feel quite right, especially around the breast area or wherever it was last found. The blue dye injected into the aureole before surgery last November has almost faded. It looks like the faint remnants of a bruise near the nipple but there is no pain connected to it. I feel around very tentatively and nervously because I'm scared I might find a lump, so while I want to check it out to assuage my fear, I don't want to search too thoroughly in case I find one.

I'm not panicking about it as next week I see my oncologist, Emma, for my scheduled visit and I can ask her if this is all right. I will also be given a thorough examination as my other two specialists have done, so I feel safe enough to wait till then.

8/10/2019 Tuesday

This traumatic experience of going through cancer and its treatments has affected me in profound ways and made me to look at myself from different angles, maybe like an artist would do. It's forced me to see myself properly and honestly and to tell the truth to myself about me. Knowing who you are is one of the most important things in life and I'm finally coming to terms with it now and can admit it without feeling embarrassed. I am a creative person. I can't live happily unless I'm creating something beautiful, interesting, unusual or just fun. I am a person who believes in being kind and I truly care about others. I feel compassion for other people in their pain and suffering. I wish everyone well; I feel pleasure in their happiness; I rejoice in their good fortune; I genuinely cheer them on to do their best. In fact, I care so much that it can come across as very weird   that's what I've learnt after hard experience. If people don't know me well enough, they tend to be suspicious about my intentions if I try to help them or empathise with them. All this doesn't mean I never get angry and sometimes feel like yelling. But then I agonise over it endlessly like I do about everything else – or have done in the past.

From now on I need to say to myself: "Don't let anyone else decide who you are. You know better than anyone who you are and if you don't like certain aspects of yourself, try to do something about it." I don't like that I'm shy – I wish I wasn't shy but I still am at sixty. Shyness has been a real scourge throughout my life stopping me from doing all sorts of things I might have been good at. I have recognised this long ago and I know now that I can't completely change it but I can accept that part of me with love instead of contempt. I need to get along with myself better and be my own best supporter first. I'm not good at technology – my mind finds it hard to take it in and remember how to work mechanical things but I can improve on using computers. I can expect myself to get better at it just like I can expect people to treat me well. I don't deserve mistreatment and rudeness and if it happens, I won't accept it. Gently but firmly, I'll stand up for myself, even if it simply means walking away and not giving that person the satisfaction of seeing me upset.

I've also come to understand that if you want to be healthy you need to change the way you talk to yourself; change the way you think about yourself; change the things you do for yourself. Change! Change! Change! – it's the real sign of life – it's the getting out of stagnation and negative patterns. Refuse to go along with other people's summary of you in the past - which means before this moment. Insults such as, "You're ugly! You're stupid! You're hopeless!" are other people's assessments all with hidden agendas to make you react in a certain limited way.

I've been called ugly at different times in my life and I believed those people who were usually insensitive, thoughtless or nasty. I didn't realise how lucky I was to have a healthy, working body that didn't give me any trouble. That I was short and freckly didn't affect that and should have been a secondary consideration, if any at all. I've relived those hurts and insults so many times, smarting at the injustice and meanness of being criticised and looked down on for things I couldn't help. So now I say to myself: Stop ruminating about the past; stop it in its tracks – say to yourself, "It's over!" and be in the moment which is usually pretty good. I can say truthfully, I have a better feeling about myself and a respect for my beautiful body I've never had before.

LIFE LESSON: TREAT YOURSELF WITH KINDNESS

Use only positive words and expressions when speaking to yourself or about yourself either mentally or out loud. Notice any negativity and stop being over-critical - show yourself the compassion you would give others. Realise that you deserve to be treated well – mostly by you! Be kind to yourself in every way and extend that loving kindness to everyone you come into contact with.

This will be a time that tests you in every way and most of all it tests your endurance to maximum capacity. You have to try and rise above every horrible thing that comes your way or it will pull you down and defeat you. Don't waste your effort thinking, "Why me?" or "It's not fair". That's a waste of time - of course it's not fair – who's arguing? - and there are people worse off than you are anyway. Letting go doesn't mean giving up. Let go of all negativity and everything that saps your energy –

all negative thoughts and habits from the past, all worries and anxiety about the future, and focus on today – on right now, on this moment. Let go of unnecessary fears and burdens that have been weighing you down because they are draining you of the little energy you have and you need every little bit of it to get to the other side of this – to get to where you can see the tiny, bright sparkle of light shining on the horizon, to get to where you feel positive about yourself and the direction you're travelling in. You've got to be facing the right way with your head full of positive thoughts and your heart open to positive outcomes. You must bring everything you have to this challenge and call on all your reserves of strength - emotional, physical and spiritual and hold on. Endure, really endure, until you get to the other side of this - until you've seen it through – until you can say, "It was dreadful, but it's over!"

9/10/2019 Wednesday

When something major happens to your body it's showing you that something's wrong and you need to make major changes to the way you're thinking and what you're doing. Having been through major illness with John we learnt this – we saw it happen to other people who had similar bypasses and lived a few short years after them. You have to change your lifestyle, your eating habits, your way of thinking about yourself and your body if you want to live. If you do the same thing that you did before, you'll end up with the same results.

I know there are many reasons why illness happens and you can spend your life getting to the bottom of it and you never will. Maybe you came into this life to experience this; maybe your body had a predisposition to this illness through your DNA and heredity; maybe it's part of aging and the body is breaking down. I don't know what the causes of cancer are, but some things I have come across ring true for me in a deep, resounding way. And I want to be honest and look at things clearly and unblinkingly and not be afraid – and not be shy about saying what I think either.

I believe that when it comes to healing you should use everything at your disposal. Some people laugh at alternative therapies such as Reiki, Crystals, Hypnotherapy and Acupuncture but you should never dismiss things you don't understand. I advocate using all the medical technology that's available to us but I also think traditional medicines have a lot to offer – and can be used to promote healing - not instead of modern medicines but as well as.

Sometimes I think: if only there could be some gem, some infinite wisdom, some shining light that sums it all up, that tells me where I've been going wrong and what I'm to do to set it straight but somehow when my mind is quiet, I know the message is so simple: rest, be happy and enjoy your life – choose what makes you feel peaceful and good; let go of all that makes you cringe and brings static and disharmony to your life. Take happiness from the present moment and make your life as simple and easy as you can. Be present for yourself and for those around you – don't always be thinking of something else or of the next thing you have to do. Just focus on what's right in front of you – on this moment – Now – and bring love to everything and mostly to yourself – because then you can spread plenty around.

Recently I have come across a great poem called, "Love after Love" by Derek Walcott, a West Indian poet. It's about welcoming into your life the stranger that is your neglected self and giving yourself the love that you so readily shower on others.

I have learnt a couple of important things over a lifetime of teaching both primary and secondary levels: be present to the children that come into your life. Say to them in your heart, "I can see you. I can hear you. You are important to me," so they don't ever have to feel invisible around you. I also do this with adults that come into my sphere now. The other thing I've learnt is the things I do are not as important as who I am. The people around you don't really care how much you know or how good you are at things; the most important thing is how you make them feel when you're around.

Stop fretting about the past - what you should have done - it's a pointless waste of energy - as for me, I've still been doing it even though I said I wouldn't years ago, but it's hard to break old habits - don't be afraid to look back but keep moving forward. Keep trying, keep pulling yourself up about it – it gets better. Each time you don't fall back as far and you pick yourself up quicker and each time you do that you can find your way ahead with more trust and confidence. Being present is important in your care of others but it's most important for your self-care.

LIFE LESSON: FOCUS ON THE NOW

You can spend a lifetime reflecting on the past and worrying about the future and neither of those things is going to give you much sense of fulfillment or satisfaction. When your mind strays into old, stressful patterns, keep bringing your thoughts back to the present. Say to yourself, "This is where I am right now and it's pretty good," - and if it isn't, change it!

12/10/2019 Saturday

The relief I felt yesterday after my appointment with Emma, my oncologist I can still feel today. Everything was normal and I am progressing well. When I asked Emma if there was anything I could do to stop the cancer recurring and to speed up my recovery she said that exercising is the best in every way and also not becoming overweight. These two things are important to good health. To sum it up, I have specifically asked about this on my follow-up visits and all three of my specialists have said similar things – exercise – especially walking, maintain a healthy weight, eat good food and remain positive. So according to the experts these are the keys to a healthy life.

17/10/2019 Thursday 8.55am

Doctor Frankel sent me to have a blood test which I've had this morning to test all the usual things. Only the left arm can be used for that because of the breast surgery on the right side. The vein in my arm which in the past was big and bold is now hard to see and the phlebotomist, Faizel, said it didn't feel like a vein. Apparently, it feels hard like a tendon because of overuse. Apart from the Chemo treatments, this would have happened because of the pneumonia and the stay in hospital which required an intravenous drip constantly pumping in the antibiotics. Breast cancer has had a detrimental effect on my body in so many unexpected ways. "The vein appears to be hiding," I said to Faizel. "It might be trying to tell me something: I think it's saying, 'No more of this! That's enough now.'" He agreed it was probably true. "It's saying, 'Keep away!'" he said, and we both had a laugh about it.

19/10/19 Saturday 2.30pm

It would have been Anthony's Birthday today. Just spoke to Vincent on the phone and he and Maria and I talked about Anthony mostly and the funny things he used to say and do. We can have a laugh about it now, which we couldn't do last year so it must mean things are getting back onto an even keel.

I remember Yvonne saying to me about three years ago when we were talking about grief that people expect you to get over it but you never do; you just have to learn to live with it – and that was very wise because it's true. Having experienced real grief herself, she knew what it meant. My brother and sister and I can actually talk about Anthony now without crying although we all miss him a lot and always will. Maybe it means things are getting back to some sort of normal.

In the last week I've been noticing an occasional hair of mine falling out which hasn't happened up till now since it started growing back months ago - every single hair has hung on tenaciously until it's become a thick mass. It shows things must be getting back to normal in my body as well.

22/10/2019 Tuesday

My doctor's appointment went well and it's clear that my health is improving. I asked Doctor Frankel about the thickening at the sides of my throat which appeared after the first Chemo treatment and have persisted until now. He wasn't too concerned about it as my blood tests showed my thyroid was fine and he said he couldn't feel any signs of a goitre – thank goodness! That hadn't even entered my thoughts. Anyway, as long as it's nothing too serious I can relax about it.

We have to see our accountant this week to get our income tax done. You can't completely avoid jobs and duties you don't particularly care to do in life, although it's lovely to see Fiona who makes things totally easy for us. We miss her uncle, Michael, who was our accountant for over thirty years until he recently died of cancer. It was always good to see him and hear his humorous take on things. Fiona told us her sister has just been through breast cancer too. I can't help agreeing with John's heart specialist, Doctor Tremain, who said it was an epidemic, as you can't mention breast cancer in particular without hearing about another person who has had it, is going through it or has died of it.

After the tax is done, John and I are going out to lunch. Now we try to make everything fun or have a fun element to it – although that's not so easy when it comes to things like sweeping the floor. I used to dance with the broom but these days my arthritic knee protests too much and my energy levels mean I can't do more than a sedate fox trot instead of the gliding waltz I used to do around the dining room.

26/10/2019 Saturday

Anthony's anniversary today – four years since he's been gone. I don't think I'll ever stop missing his physical presence, after all, he was my caring brother for fifty-five years. Not so much despite this but because of this and seeing how hard he was striving till the last moment to make everything better in his life, I need to acknowledge and accept that I've had a lucky escape and it strengthens my resolution to make this second chance I've been given, the happiest time of my life. I feel a bit weather beaten and tired like old Josephine, our visiting magpie, with her slightly dragging wing and ruffled plumage but still singing, regardless of setting or circumstance, because I am hopeful that the best is yet to come.

What a superb spring day this is! I find that I'm enjoying the garden even more than before and appreciating the magnificence of nature and what an astounding gift it is. The blackbirds love the front yard, hopping in and out of the violet patch and the honeyeaters are delighting in the bottlebrushes and grevillea. The flowering crab apple is looking the most spectacular it's ever been - green and covered in buds ready to burst, full of such beauty and promise. All of it fills me with renewed hope about the next phase of my life.

28/10/2019 Monday

The lilacs are in bloom and they are gorgeous, spreading their sweet fragrance around the front yard and in through the bedroom window. I don't think they've ever been so glorious. The freesias are still flowering and sending out their exquisite scent. The garden looks magnificent, green and lush and full of life, with splashes of colourful spring bulbs here and there. The two Peace roses are superb – all golden and edged with deep pink. The flowering crab apple is covered in voluptuous pink and white blossoms and buzzing with the musical hum of hundreds of bees. All the sounds, perfumes and colours are so vivid and real.

Physically I feel fine: my eyesight is back to normal; my balance has returned; I have my sense of smell again and I am delighting in being surrounded by nature - the ultimate affirmation of life. Months ago, I hoped this could happen and my wish has come true. It feels like a reawakening of all my senses and my enjoyment of everything has been heightened because of it. I love this moment - in the garden just outside the bedroom window - and I'm actually looking forward to tomorrow.

31/10/2019 Thursday

I definitely feel I'm getting better every day and feeling better about myself as my body heals and I am past the worst and scariest parts of dealing with surgery, Chemotherapy and Radiation treatment. I have gone through it – I have endured the triple negative phase of my life and I am beginning to feel physically well again and mentally stronger than ever before. The great skill and care of all the medical experts, the love of all the people around me and my own resolve have got me through and I'm determined more than ever to make the most of this second chance. The cancer has been eradicated and with it the harmful, self-destructive thoughts that kept telling me I wasn't good enough.

7/11/2019

Have caught up with my friend Jill today and to see her was like a breath of fresh air. She looked tanned and healthy and was catching up with quite a few friends while she and her husband, Malcolm, had come back to Melbourne for six weeks. They have been touring around Australia in a big caravan for the last two years and are going for at least two more. She has come to the conclusion that our houses are full of things we don't need and are then forced to look after, and intends to scale down after their trip is over. As I listen happily to the interesting stories about the small forgotten towns they have visited and the friendliness and hospitality of the people, it acts like a restorative balm to me. Jill's on a grand adventure which, to her own surprise, she is enjoying immensely. The other surprise she has experienced is the huge change which has happened in some of her friends' lives over the two short years she has been away: two have been widowed and two have contracted breast cancer and to my own continuing disbelief, I am one of the latter. She has just visited another friend who has been through her first Chemo treatment and has been coping valiantly. It doesn't matter who I'm speaking to, this topic of breast cancer in the last recent years seems to have become part of everyone's sphere of experience in one way or another.

8/11/2019

Saw an amazing news story about cancer research – huge advancement is occurring. Australian scientists have discovered a virus that blasts all cancer cells and is working well in mice. The human trials will begin next year when they will target Triple Negative breast cancer first. I'm thinking that maybe because it's the most aggressive. This is also great news because we don't have to wait years for results the way things used to be. These results could make a difference in my own lifetime and perhaps in a few short years or sooner, Chemotherapy could become obsolete. That would be a truly great day.

12/11/2019

The rainbow lorikeets are chirruping happily high up in the trees along our back fence. Their orange-gold breasts and bright green wings make them look like flowers from where I'm standing below them in the garden, and as I look up through the branches that make a pattern against the blue, their azure heads are just that colour of the sky. You wouldn't think such colourful birds could be so camouflaged but in among the branches of the Silky Oaks which are full of feathery green leaves and golden flower combs, the lorikeets blend in magnificently and can't be distinguished unless they move. They don't mind me at all and continue with their preening and playfulness. I look at them with a sense of awe, feeling I am part of their sociable, chatty group, free from all worries and anxieties.

18/11/2019

It's the morning of my mammogram and ultrasound tests before I see my surgeon for my end of treatment check-up next week. This has been looming on the calendar for a while for me and I've felt in two minds about it: I'm sort of dreading it but at the same time I want to have them done so that I can be certain there are no signs of cancer.

"I'm sorry you have to go through all this," says John. "It's horrible." I haven't spoken about it but John obviously knows how I feel. "Don't worry," I reassure him, "As long as the results are good, I don't mind," I add, feeling much more worried than I'm letting on. I've had some pain, particularly in my right breast occasionally during the last months so I have a feeling of uncertainty and nervousness about the tests and results. In fact, I'm surprised at how nervous I'm feeling this morning.

When we arrive at the clinic, providentially I'm called in almost at once and the mammogram is quickly under way with Patricia who is efficient and gentle. The procedure is very uncomfortable as my breasts feel tender – but it's quick. The ultrasound is done shortly after, starting with the left breast. At times it's quite painful which makes me ask Ragavi, the sonographer, "Is this normal?" She says no but adds that some women are very sensitive in the breast area and I admit I'm one of them.

After it's over Ragavi tells me it looks all right. I'm so glad she has let me know this as last time I was told nothing until I saw my own G.P. She says that a doctor will examine the results and then the scans will be given to me before I leave but there should be nothing to worry about according to the ultrasound I've just had. I am so relieved and grateful that I thank her many times for letting me know.

I tell John about it in the waiting room and we both feel confident that if the tests had shown any problems I would be told to go and see my G.P. today and as none of that is happening, I can feel almost certain it's all clear and I can relax.

One really tough thing about surviving cancer is having to live with the uncertainty that every ache and every pain might be the cancer returning. It can take over your life if you're not careful. I want to make sure that after I've had the check-up with my specialist, I get rid of these thoughts and feelings that can ruin my peace of mind. I have to accept that it's one of those fears that's common and normal for anyone who's had cancer and kick those thoughts right out of my head as soon as they try to sneak in. I think I'll even say it with the words: "Get out!" like I would to a pesky fly buzzing around my kitchen – then add after a bit: "And stay out!"

John and I drive off from the MRI Clinic rejoicing and I'm feeling a sense of euphoria mixed with a tiny bit of doubt and tons of tiredness all at once. I think the tiredness is from the tension that's been building up over the last few days knowing the tests were coming up – and which I'd suppressed. The bit of doubt is maybe going to always be there but all that doesn't matter now. I'm okay and that's all that counts. We can go home and celebrate with a few phone calls to people we love.

26/11/2019

Today was the day of days. This morning I saw Julia, my surgeon who looked at the mammogram and ultrasound images and said everything was looking good. Consequently, I don't need to see her for another year. It was such great news that I'm still revelling in it.

The pain that happens intermittently in my right breast is also okay and normal for what it's been through apparently, so that was good news too. I am elated and feel really relieved – I can't express how relieved. I can really start to let go of this hideous anxiety that's been sneakily hiding at the back of my mind and weighing heavily on me. It feels like a heavy burden has been lifted away and now I can breathe easier. Everything is looking very positive for me now and I can expect a full recovery and more time enjoying this beautiful world and all the wonderful people I've been blessed to have in my life.

31/12/2019

It's hard to believe this is the last day of 2019. What a crazy year it's been! But I'm still here to talk about it. I'm still standing at the end of it as I hoped I'd be. All that illness *was* just temporary and I'm okay – actually better than okay – and looking forward to all the good things to come. The Chinese Star Jasmine along the driveway has almost finished flowering. It was planted before we moved in and is not what we would have chosen to plant along the path but it has proved to be perfect exactly where it is. Its delicate fragrance fills the front yard for weeks year after year and the small white flowers are not obvious but stunning when you notice them. Its perfume is rivalled only by the mauve Buddleia we have transplanted with us every time we have shifted house. It's Dad's plant – he planted a cutting more than thirty years ago and it's come with us to each new garden.

Tomorrow is the start of a brand new year and a brand new way of living. Good-bye to all the aches and pains and hurts of the last twelve months! I will treasure and bring with me all that's good from the past and let everything else go. It has been the most testing and difficult time of my life, but I've come through it more grateful than ever for my beautiful life, my husband, my family and my friends and I'm looking forward to the amazing and wonderful experiences to come that are part of being alive.

August the Following Year 24/8/2020 Monday

This morning I was the only one in the small lift at Cabrini Hospital making my way down to the car after my appointment with Emma, my oncologist for my four-monthly check-ups. John had gone ahead to pay the parking at the ticket machine. I was still smiling and feeling relieved and happy that I'd received a good report about my progress, when a woman a few years older than me got into the lift at the next level. She was taller than me and had an imposing presence, but she looked hassled and worn out with fairly messy hair – and she came in coughing. I glanced at her a bit alarmed. I've been very wary of strangers with sniffles or coughs since this pandemic started. She must have read my thoughts. "Don't worry it's not Covid," she said, without looking at me, "I'm having Chemo." My expression was suddenly very serious. I nodded, understanding exactly what she meant. I could see she felt rotten and she'd had enough. Her whole body seemed fidgety and she sounded frustrated and bitter. "I went through it last year," I said simply. She looked at me then. "So, you can get through it!" she said, half angrily. "Yes, you *can* get through it," I repeated earnestly, and then the lift stopped and she was out and gone. I didn't get a chance to say anything more, such as, "Hold on! Don't give up! It'll get better." But maybe none of that was necessary. She had heard all anyone going through it needs to know: "You can get through it."

October One Year Later 1/10/2021 Friday

I've sent that lady many good wishes from my heart since then, as I've done for all the other cancer patients I've met along the way who were having similar treatments. That incident in the lift lasted only a few moments but there was one really positive thing about it for me: it was obvious that I looked like an ordinary, healthy person. I have never wanted the cancer to define me – my life is much more than that and I want to learn from the experience and move on from it.

So, now that I'm enjoying this new phase of my life, I wish you all good health and happiness, especially those of you who have had a diagnosis of cancer. Lean on the help and love of others even if you have never done that before; surround yourself with caring, loving people; rely on your medical team; acknowledge to yourself that what you're going through is terrible, and then think positive thoughts about getting well. Bring everything you've got to this experience, especially patience, because you're going to need it and just know – You can get through it.

Now it's just over two years since the end of my treatments and not only do I look well, I am well. It's clear that I am back to good health - in fact with a far healthier attitude and a happier outlook and feeling better about myself than ever before. This year one of my dreams has already been fulfilled: my three children's books have finally been published and are out in the world and that gives me a feeling of genuine happiness.

This life is golden and I don't want to waste another moment thinking I need to be something else – constantly striving to be better in some way – it's exhausting! I just need to get on with being myself. I've always wished everyone well. Now I extend that good will to me and allow myself to be peaceful - and not to feel guilty or apologetic ever again for being sad if that's how I feel - or joyful, successful and happy in the things that are important to me.

This arduous journey has made me see everything from a different perspective: I feel I know myself better; I can accept all the good that comes to me; I know I can hold my ground among equals; now, finally I own my space. And as soon as I catch myself going down a path full of negative thoughts, I say to myself, "Turn around – you're going the wrong way!"

No more Triple Negative for me – only Positive! Positive! Positive!

Afterword

It's coming up to four years since the end of my treatment and I know I am getting better all the time. I've had to be patient though and I still experience some fatigue but there are many positive things that have come out of this horrible experience of having breast cancer. I have learnt to be much kinder to myself and not push too hard. I still get things done but I don't mind if I take longer to do them or if I change my mind and not do some things at all. I am much more flexible and relaxed about everything now and I take time to enjoy life. I am more in tune with what makes me happy. It has also made me understand the fear associated with serious illness from a very personal perspective and helped me to be even more empathetic and compassionate towards anyone going through it.

Looking back, if I had to summarise what I learned from my experience – and am still learning – it's that life really is so short and so precious. One of the most important things that going through breast cancer has taught me is to enjoy the here and now – just be fully present wherever you are and you'll be continually reminded that life is good: reflect on the past and learn from it; think about the future and look forward to it, but focus on the now and enjoy every moment. At the start of each day say to yourself, "This is a new beginning for me."

I offer you my very best wishes for your healing and recovery and for complete well-being.

With love from, Grace Nolan.

A Few Extras

Grace's Waterfall Meditation

This is a meditation which I have made up and used throughout the treatments and it has really helped me. I lie down or sit in a comfortable chair and then I usually read this and visualise it, taking deep, steady breaths:

I am under a beautiful, healing waterfall. Mild, cool, crystal-clear water is pouring gently onto my head and running down my neck, arms and body, down my hips and legs, over my knees and down to my toes, washing away with it all heat and discomfort from my body; washing away all toxins and pain, washing away everything that no longer serves me, clearing away all heaviness and illness, clearing away all unnecessary fears, clearing away all feelings of stress; refreshing and cleansing me as it pours down in a soft, pure, steady stream, revitalising me, replenishing me; restoring me to good health and peace of mind, healing me in all ways: physically, spiritually, emotionally, mentally and intellectually; giving me calmness, coolness, balance and beauty. And with every heartbeat, with every breath, the healing continues for as long as I need it.

Jan's Healing Meditation

Lorrie sent this to me from her friend, Jan, in Wales. I have loved using it as a meditation, visualising myself in the way Jan describes but changing the water to cool instead of tepid as I have felt too hot throughout the treatments.

I visualise myself in a gentle running stream in the forest. There is nothing there that can harm me – not a thorn or insect or any creepy crawly. The water is very gentle on my skin; it is tepid and very clear as it comes from upstream - it is crystal clear. As it passes me it changes colour, because all worries, pains, cancer cells and feelings of tiredness wash away.

Some foods and recipes
that helped me feel better during Chemo:-

- Boiled eggs sliced into a sandwich or in a roll or on their own with salt

- Pasta with peas (peas can be frozen or fresh)

- Pasta with beans (beans can be dry and soaked overnight or tinned)

- Vegetable soup

- Avocado with mayonnaise in a roll, sandwich or Salada biscuit

- Smoked tuna roll with mayonnaise

- Fish fillets fried or baked with steamed vegetables (pour gravy over top of veg if liked)

- Plain roast chicken with baked vegetables

- Sizzle steak very thin and fried quickly

- Plain Weeties – leave them to sit in skim milk and a little sugar to soften them up. After I've eaten the Weeties I throw out the left over milk in the bowl

- Porridge

- Scrambled eggs

- Toast

- Blueberries, strawberries and cherries in the first weeks then found they caused too much indigestion

- Boiling water in a cup with 3 small pieces of raw ginger in it (instead of tea)

- Keep all foods plain with no pepper or paprika – just salt and maybe herbs if liked

- Golden Circle cordials are good for drinking – keep them in fridge and mix them with tap water so drink isn't too cold

I found it best to avoid all food and drink that's too hot or cold, such as hot tea, ice cream – as it gave me a stomach ache and I felt sick with it for hours. Things out of the fridge were fine to eat such as fruit but I had to leave them out for a bit. I could have nothing straight out of the freezer – it was too cold.

The following two recipes are based on the Southern Italian peasant food passed down to my mother and then to my sister and me.

Recipe for Pasta and Peas

INGREDIENTS

- 1 carrot
- 1 onion
- 1 potato
- ½ cup Italian passata (tomato sauce)
- 3 tablespoons olive oil
- Salt
- 500 grams peas (frozen or fresh)

METHOD

1. In a medium saucepan -
2. Dice carrot, onion and potato
3. Fry in the oil for a couple of minutes
4. Add peas and fry for another three minutes
5. Add 1/2 a cup of passata - Italian tomato sauce and cook for further 5 minutes
6. Add water and salt to taste and bring to boil
7. Simmer gently for 15-20 minutes
8. Add pasta – ditalini or paternosti is perfect for this – or any sort desired
9. Cook till pasta is ready – about 10-15 minutes
10. Add a little more water and salt if needed

Recipe for Pasta and Beans

INGREDIENTS

- A couple of handfuls of dry beans – borlotti, cannellini or any type of dry beans
- Tinned beans can be used instead to save time and effort
- 1 tomato
- 1 potato
- 1 onion
- 5 broccoli florets or a couple of leaves of silver beet (optional)
- Salt
- Spaghetti

METHOD

1. Put a couple of handfuls of dry beans into a bowl and cover with water to soak overnight

2. Next day drain water and place the beans in a saucepan with fresh water and salt

3. Add one diced tomato, one diced potato and one diced onion

4. Add small piece of diced pumpkin if desired

5. Add steamed broccoli or silver beet if desired

6. When beans and other ingredients are soft add the spaghetti

7. Cook till spaghetti is al dente

8. This dish can be as brothy or as thick as you like by adding more or less water and salt as desired

9. An onion can be fried in a little olive oil first which gives a different flavour to the dish

Acknowledgements

I thank with sincerest gratitude my husband John and my family and friends: Maria, Vincent, Lorrie, Grace, Vince, Sandy, Pauline, Paul, Bridgette, Ryan, Gail, Cameron, Renee, Daniel, Deana, Alexia, Michael P, Steven P, Nea, Norm, Ann, Ron, Moira, Yvonne, Steven R, Rozanne, Janine, Joy, Rodrigo, Jill, Malcolm, Bill, Paulineke, Cathy, Paul, Michael S, Megan, David, Sonia, Allison, Hailey, Caitlin, Sarah, Beau, Heath, Abel, Isla, Aidan, Kaycee, Melina, Anne G, Ian, Dzintra, Francis, Jan M, Harold, Anne T, Kim, Greg, Tony, Karen A, Melinda, Neil, Jenella, Lorraine, Jenny, Elton, Jan A, Heather, Fiona and my medical team, Mark, Sarah K, Lara, Karen T, Warwick and Peter.

Thank you to PublishMyBook.Online, especially James Munro, for your patience and expertise in transforming my manuscript into this published book.

Other Books by Grace Nolan

A set of three counting books for young children introducing counting to 10 in Book 1, adding to 10 in Book 2 and subtracting from 10 in Book 3.

Published 2021 by Big Sky Publishing.

Book 1: *10 Naughty Numbats*

Book 2: *10 Bush Babies*

Book 3: *10 Lively Lorikeets*

Website: www.gracenolanauthor.com

Facebook: Grace Nolan Author